Intermittent Fasting for Women

Little-Known Secrets for Weight Loss and Burn Fat in a Fast and Easy Way, Discover the Metabolic Process of Autophagy and Improve Your Life Quality

Dr. Jason Stephens

publisher for any reparation, damages, or monetary loss due to the information herein, either directly or indirectly.

Respective authors own all copyrights not held by the publisher.

The information herein is offered for informational purposes solely, and is universal as so. The presentation of the information is without contract or any type of guarantee assurance.

The trademarks that are used are without any consent, and the publication of the trademark is without permission or backing by the trademark owner. All trademarks and brands within this book are for clarifying purposes only and are the owned by the owners themselves, not affiliated with this document

Table of content

Introduction

You may have heard of the positive effects of fasting for the body. It not only helps you to lose weight; it also makes your mind better and gives you greater energy. But where do you start?

As a woman your physiology is different from that of a man and the chapters below will cover all you need to learn to get going with intermittent fasting. This is a great diet plan which focuses more on the time to eat foods than the actual food you eat. There are also a wide range of options when it comes to using the intermittent fast so that you can make it work for your lifestyle.

This book gives you all the details you need to get started with an intermittent fast. We'll look at what's all about this easy, the health benefits that come with it, how to eat on this diet plan, and more.

You are going to learn the ins and outs of fasting. How you apply this information is up to you. Maybe you want to set a daily fasting timetable, or maybe you want to fast spontaneously, when the moment is driving you. You might want to lose weight as well as tackle health problems.

Whatever your motivations for intermittent fasting are, this book is here to help you embrace this new lifestyle with courage and adapt it to your life— easily and effectively.

Chapter 1

Intermittent fasting, as the name implies, is a practice in which you routinely go on without food. This doesn't mean that you're hungry-far from it. Rather, you mix fasting with a healthy diet, becoming mindful of what you are eating and drinking to promote better fitness and clarity of mind. Intermittent fasting will help you tackle diabetes and other disorders associated with high blood sugar, as well as everything from insomnia to heart disease, if you do it in the right way. If you are interested in intermittent fasting, the details below will help you get started.

What Is Intermittent Fasting?

Intermittent fasting consists of a dieter alternating between times where food is permitted and a period when fasting is supposed to take place. This type of diet does not necessarily say which foods to consume, but determines when to feed. For example, eating foods that are healthier for you and nutritious is ideal if you want to lose weight or get better health. For intermittent fasting, though, it won't specifically mention which things you can and can't have.

There are different types of sporadic methods of fasting, but they all break the day or week into feeding hours and fasting cycles. What you might be surprised to know is that when we eat, most of us are still fasting every day. You might be able to extend the normal fast time a bit further. You may decide to skip breakfast, for example, and have your first meal at midday and your last meal at 8 pm. That would be seen as a form of intermittent fasting.

You technically fast for up for sixteen hours each day with this approach and then feed only during an eight-hour period of the day. This mode of fasting is one of the common options when it comes to intermittent fasting, also known as the 16/8 process.

Despite what you might think right now, intermittent fasting is very easy. It doesn't take a lot of planning and countless people who've been on this diet say they feel better and have more energy when on a fast. You may struggle with hunger in the beginning, but it won't take long before your body adapts and becomes used to it.

The main thing to remember is that you are not allowed to eat when you're in a period of fasting. Beverages can still be consumed to keep you hydrated. Some of the choices are tea, coffee, soda, and other non-calorie beverages. Many aspects of this fast during the fasting cycles can allow for a bit of food, but most don't. And if you like, taking a drink is usually fine while you're on this easy, as long as it doesn't contain calories.

A History of Fasting

Easy, daily access to food is actually a fairly new concept when it comes to society culture. People had to rely solely on the soil to get food before the Industrial Revolution. We just could not take a ride to their nearest grocery store if we needed to fill their stomachs. Ancient civilizations (and some today's world civilizations) hunted and harvested as much as they could, but food was not always a guarantee. Sometimes the hunters and gatherers would come back with a fresh kill and load of fresh fruits and berries; other days would come back empty-handed, especially in times of drought such as the winter months.

While they did not do it deliberately, these days they were practically fasting. Such fasts might last days, weeks, or even months, depending on the time of year and the abilities of the hunters and gatherers.

Apart from this forced fasting, some ancient cultures got on to the benefits of fasting well before modern research. The ancient Greeks believed that fasting could enhance your focus and cognitive abilities. Benjamin Franklin, one of America's founding fathers, and the alleged inventor of lightning rod and bifocal lenses, wrote, "Resting and fasting is the greatest of all medicines."

Spiritual Fasting

Fasting was–and is –also an important part of different beliefs and spiritual practices around the world. Fasting is often defined as a healing or purification method when used for religious purposes, but the basic concept remains the same: abstain from eating for a given period of time.

Unlike therapeutic fasting, which is used as a cancer cure, spiritual fasting is seen as a significant tool for the health of the whole body, and a wide range of religions hold the idea that fasting has the power to heal. Fasting in Buddhism is a way of exercising abstinence from acting on human desires, a discipline which Buddhist monks consider to be a piece of the puzzle to achieving nirvana. Most Buddhists fast every day, eating food in the morning then abstaining from feeding for the remainder of the day until the next morning is time to eat. Besides this, the Buddhists also embark for days or weeks on a water-only fast.

Fasting in Christianity is a way to cleanse the spirit in order to make the body sacred and to create a bond with God. The forty-day period between Ash Wednesday and Easter is one of the most popular times that Christians fast is called Lent. Those who followed Lent gave up food or drink in earlier days; in more modern times, Christians may still abstain from food and drink, but they often prefer to go without a specific thing. This custom is supposed to be an indication of the forty days Jesus Christ was compelled to fast in the wilderness.

Within Hinduism it is believed that by fasting, ignoring the body's physical needs helps to increase spirituality. While fasting is a regular part of the Hindu religion and is often practiced, one of the most famous fasts performed is during Maha Shivaratri, or the "Great Night of Shiva." During Maha Shivaratri, devotees fast, take part in ceremonial baths, visit a temple where they pray, and exercise the virtues of loyalty, pardon, and self-discipline.

There are several explanations for fasting in Judaism, including calling for God's grace, remembering important life events, expressing reverence to God, or mourning; however, keeping the fast secret is customary when you do a person fast.

Within Mormonism there is a tradition called Fast Sunday, in which adherents on the first Sunday of each month abstain from two meals (for a total of twenty-four hours). Members share personal experiences with their church community during this fast, in an extra effort to cleanse and purify. They frequently contribute to the church the equivalent cost of these two meals to help the needy — a practice known as a fast donation.

Perhaps a feature of the Muslim religion is the most well-known holy fast, Ramadan. During Ramadan, not only do Muslims abstain from dusk to dawn from food and drink but they also avoid smoking, sexual intercourse, and any other practices that may be considered immoral. The fasting period— and the slight starvation that happens due to lack of fluids— is thought to cleanse the mind from unhealthy impurities so that the conscience can be turned to salvation and away from earthly desires.

These are of course only a few of the faiths that include fasting in their worship. Baha'i, Jainism, Sikhism, Taoism, Anglicanism, Methodism, Pentecostalism, Lutheranism, and Catholicism are other denominations that include fasting.

Medical Fasting

Hippocrates, who was given the nickname "The Father of Medicine," introduced fasting as a medical therapy for some of his sick patients as far back as the fifth century B.C.E. One of the famous quotes from Hippocrates says, "Eating when you're sick is feeding your disease." He believed that fasting allowed the body to concentrate on healing itself, and that forcing food in a sick state might actually lead to disease. On the other hand, if sick patients abstained from food, digestive processes would be shut down and natural healing would be given priority to the body.

Some of these medicinal fasts only required water and calorie-free tea for up to a month while others allowed patients to eat 200–500 calories a day. Usually the calories come from bread, broths, fruits, and milk. The specificities of the fast depended on the state of the individual.

Nevertheless, it wasn't until the 1900s that fasting began to appear as an important medical therapy for obesity and other ailments in scientific journals; even then, it wasn't until more recently that the effects completely caught on.

Why fast?

The next question you might have is why, should you consider fasting? Human beings have been going through cycles of fasting for many years. Sometimes they have done this because it was a need because they couldn't find enough food to eat. Then there were occasions when the fasting was performed for religious reasons as well. Religions like Buddhism,

Christianity, and Islam consider any sort of fasting compulsory. Fasting when you're feeling sick is natural too.

Although there is sometimes a negative connotation about fasting, there is really nothing unhealthy about fasting. Our bodies are generally well-equipped to handle occasions when we must go without food. Inside the body there are quite a few processes that shift when we are moving on a fast. This helps our bodies continue to function in times of famine.

We get a significant reduction in the levels of insulin and blood sugar as well as a dramatic rise in what is known as the human growth hormone, while we fast. While this was originally something that was done when food was scarce, it is now used to help people lose weight. Burning fat is smoother, faster, and more efficient with fasting.

Some people choose to go on a fast as this can improves their metabolism. This fasting is ideal for curing different health conditions and diseases. Interestingly, there's some evidence showing how intermittent fasting will help you live longer. Studies show that rodents with intermittent fasting were able to extend their life span.

Fasting can help protect against various diseases such as Alzheimer's disease, cancer, type-2 diabetes, and heart disease. And then there are those who choose to go on an irregular easy, because their lifestyle makes it convenient.

Fasting can be a truly effective shortcut to life. The fewer dishes you have to prepare, for example, the easier your life is.

Why does intermittent fasting work?

Intermittent fasting is the practice of planning your meals so that your body can make the most of them. Instead of slashing your calorie intake by half, depriving yourself of all the things you love, or plunging into a new diet fad, intermittent fasting is an easy, rational and safe way to eat that encourages fat loss. There are many ways to approach intermittent fasting, but it is characterized as a specific pattern of eating. Instead of what you consume, this approach relies on adjusting your feeding.

You'll more likely keep your calorie intake the same when you start intermittent fasting, but instead of spacing your meals throughout the day, you'll consume larger meals in a shorter time frame. For example, instead of consuming 3 or 4 meals a day, you could consume one big meal at 11 a.m., then another big meal at 6 p.m., with no meals between 11 a.m. and 6 p.m., and no meals before 11 a.m. the next day, after 6 p.m. This is only one intermittent fasting process, and more will be discussed in later chapters in this book. But first you have to explain why this method works.

Intermittent fasting is a technique that bodybuilders, runners, and fitness gurus use to keep their muscle mass up and their amount of body fat small. It's a simple strategy that allows you to eat the food you enjoy while still promoting fat loss and gaining or maintaining your muscles. Short-term or long-term intermittent fasting may be practiced, but the best results are from implementing this approach in your everyday lifestyle.

While the word "fasting" may cause the average person to be frightened, intermittent fasting does not mean hunger. To understand the principles behind effective intermittent fasting, first we will go over the two digestive states of the body: the fed state and the fasting state.

Your body is in what is known as the "fed state" for three to five hours after eating a meal. During the fed state, your insulin levels increase to absorb and digest the food. Burning fat is very difficult for your body when the insulin levels are high. Insulin is a protein that the pancreas generates to control blood stream glucose levels. Although it is meant to control, insulin is a storage hormone scientifically. Your body burns your food for energy when insulin levels are high, rather than your stored fat, which is why increased levels of it prevent weight loss.

Your body has finished eating the food after the three to five hours are over, and you are reaching the post-absorptive period. The post-absorbent period lasts from 8 to 12 hours everywhere. After this time gap is when your body enters the fasted state. With your body absorbing your diet fully by this stage, your insulin levels are low, making your stored fat highly accessible for burning.

In the fasted state, the body does not have any food left to use for nutrition, so instead it consumes the stored fat. Intermittent fasting helps the body to enter an advanced fat burning state you cannot usually attain with the average eating pattern of' three meals per day.' This aspect alone is why many people notice dramatic improvements of intermittent fasting without even adjusting their exercise routines, how much they sleep, or what they consume. They just change the timing and rhythm of their dietary intake.

It may take you some time to get into the swing of things when you undertake an intermittent fasting programme. Don't be deterred! When you slip up, when you can, just get back into your intermittent fasting routine. Do not beat yourself up, or feel guilty. Negative self-talk only prolongs your return to trend. It takes a concerted effort to make a lifestyle change and no one wants you to do it perfectly right away. If you're not used to going for long periods without feeding, start are used to extended fasting. You'll get the hang of it in no time as long as you choose the right method for you, stay focused and stay positive.

Unlike some of the other diet plans you can continue with, the intermittent fast is one that will work. It uses your body to its advantage, and how it works to help you really lose weight.

When you hear about fasting it's easy to get a little scared. You can think you need to go days and weeks without eating (and who's really willing to give up their diet for that long even when they want to lose weight) and it's going to be too tough for you.

Intermittent fasting is a little different from what you would expect. Not only is it painful to go on a fast at a time for weeks, but it's not good for the body, either. When you end up being on the fast for too long, your body will often go into starvation mode. This means you're in a period without a lot of food, so the body can try to save the calories and help you keep the fat and calories as long as possible. It means you're not only starving, but also lack weight loss.

You don't have to think too much about how in starvation mode this intermittent fast will work. The intermittent fast is successful because you won't run for so long that the body goes into this state of malnutrition and prevents weight loss. Instead, it will make the short last just long enough to speed up the metabolism.

With the intermittent fast, you will find that the body will not go straight into starvation mode when you go for a few hours without eating (usually no more than 24ish hours). Instead it will consume the available calories. When you eat the right amount of calories for the day, the body will be going back to eating up the remaining fat reserves and using it as food. As such, you push your body to burn more fat without putting in any extra work, whether you pursue an intermittent fasting schedule.

Here are just a few quick tips for success:

First and foremost, it's important not to expect immediate benefits from your new lifestyle. Instead, you need to plan to commit to the process for at least 30 days before you can start assessing the results accurately.

Furthermore, it is important to bear in mind that the quality of the food you put into your body also matters, as it will take only a few fast food meals to ruin all your hard work.

Finally, you'll want to throw in a moderate exercise routine for fast days and a more conventional full-calorie routine for the best results.

How Our Modern Diet is Failing Us

We all know we need healthier eating. We do realize we need to reduce our intake of alcohol, fruit, processed foods, sugars. But even though we know these things are important, it doesn't mean it's as easy to follow.

According to a recent food and health survey conducted by Psychology Today, 52 percent of Americans believe that figuring out their taxes is easier for them than figuring out how to eat healthily. Many people have trouble with the current tax code, which means that even more people find it difficult to figure out how to eat a diet that is good for them.

The world is fighting an obesity war. Less than one percent of the U.S. population is considered obese, and many are still considered overweight. Such numbers, though, do not show the full picture. Two out of three Americans are considered overweight or obese, which means more people are going to fall into this category.

Why are the statistics so dismal? There are many factors contributing to obesity. The standard human diet is one big culprit. The quality of our diets has been greatly reduced as we went from a people that relied on food from local farms to a people that mass-produces most of our food. This transition has increased our food consumption, as it's now available so readily.

Furthermore, many readily available, easy-to-eat foods are high in fat, sugars, and calories. These all lead to weight gain. From the sugary snacks we find in the break room to all the fast food chains around us, the quality of the food and the amount we eat has dramatically changed. If we wish we can literally eat non-stop unhealthy foods, which is why obesity is so prevalent in our culture.

The first thing that we should be looking at is the amount of food we consume. The amount of calories each person needs varies from individual to individual. The considerations are your ethnicity, level of activity, overall health, height, age and gender. The average figure used on food labels, though, is around 2000 calories every day. For those who lead a sedentary life this figure is already fairly high. You can also eat 2000 or more calories in just one sitting, if you go out to eat.

While eating out quickly pushes us past calorie limits, more can also be eaten even when eating at home. It's important to learn how to start eating what we need to work, rather than eating because something tastes good or we are bored, tired or sad.

In order to calculate the total amount of daily calories consumed, organizations are analyzing the amount of food available per person as measures of how much food is eaten. It ends up being about 3800 calories per day inside the U.S. Even if you compensate for some of this food being lost or dumped every day rather than eaten, the American population only eats 2700 calories every day. That's much more than anyone will need, even if they live an active lifestyle that many People don't.

However, we also need to think about the quality of the food that we consume. As we grow up, most of us learn from our parents and teachers which food is good and which is not. Fruits and vegetables are considered good, and desserts and sugars are evil. The rest of the food might not have been as healthy for you but in balance they were perfect. And though we've been educated about healthy eating at a young age, in reality, following this recommendation is much more difficult.

According to the U.S. The top six calorie sources for most Americans in the Department of Agriculture are grain-based foods, yeast bread, chicken, soda/sports and health drinks, and alcoholic beverages. Remember that organic fruits and vegetables do not appear on the list. Most of the foods that Americans consume are refined grains and sugars. Just 8 per cent of America's average diet is estimated to consist of fruits and vegetables.

According to a 2010 report by the U.S. Department of Agriculture (USDA), grains, proteins and eggs make up 21% of those diets; sugar and fat make up 23% and caloric sweeteners make up 15%. The food which is not so good for us makes up 61 percent of our diets.

The time of day we eat also matters. Most people live a busy lifestyle, and have no time to sit down and eat a well-balanced meal. They feed on the go, usually at some unhealthy place, or they eat at night because their metabolisms are sluggish. Furthermore, when watching TV, many people sit on the couch and eat unhealthy snack foods. The food tastes so good that we eat it non-stop.

It's important to learn the steps necessary to limit the amount of food we eat each day. Eating foods which are readily available is enticing. But if you want to restore your health and stay in good condition, it's crucial to move away from the typical diet and choose something better and healthier for you.

You may think of people who go for weeks without eating for religious reasons, when you hear about fasting. You may think its bad, or because you love food too much, you won't be able to do so. Yet intermittent fasting is distinct from traditional fasting though some common concepts are exchanged.

Intermittent fasting is about restricting the calorie intake or not eating as much on certain days during certain times of the day. The body always receives the nutrients it needs so you eat fewer calories, making weight loss harder.

The reason this diet is popular is because it is effective in reducing both the amount of fat in your body and the number of calories you eat. Since you're limiting the time frame you're allowed to eat or reduce the calorie intake over certain days of the week, it's much better to lower the overall calorie count.

You can also choose how long the sporadic easy you'd like to do. Many people want to do it for a month or so while others suit it in their lives, and they stick with it for a long time to come.

What is obesity and what causes it?

Obesity is a complex disease that involves an unhealthy amount of body fat. It is a medical condition that increases the chances of having other diseases and health problems, such as heart disease, diabetes, high blood pressure and certain cancers.

There are a variety of reasons why some women are having difficulty preventing obesity. Typically, obesity is the result of a combination of genetic causes, along with the environment and personal diet and exercise choices.

Good news is that even moderate weight loss will boost or avoid obesity-related health problems. Dietary changes, increased physical activity and behavioral changes will help you lose weight. Prescription medications and weight-loss treatments are potential choices for the treatment of obesity.

What Causes Obesity?

Obesity can be complex. You gain weight because you eat more calories than you work out. Yet the weight may be affected by certain variables. They include;

1.What and how you eat.

In today's culture, consuming unhealthy foods and over-eating is easy. Many things, including emotions, habits, and access to food, can influence eating behavior.

2.How active are you

New conveniences— like elevators, vehicles, and television remote control— try and avoid such conveniences. Being active helps you stay fit and healthy. You burn more calories when you're fit, even if you're sleeping.

3.Your genetic makeup

The impact of your genetic makeup on your weight is very high. It affects;

- The rate, at which the body uses energy (calories) during a rest, is called the basal metabolic rate. Many people are born with higher metabolic baseline levels than others. They burn more calories, of course, than others.

- You can increase your metabolic rate through regular physical activity.

- Low-calorie foods are going to lower the metabolic rate. If you don't burn calories as quickly, a high metabolic rate makes it easier to gain weight.

- Signals from your body, like your hunger, feeling hungry or full.

- Distribution of your fat. You have no control on how your body stores fat. Women hold more fat in the hips and thighs. When women age, the belly accumulates more fat.

4.A diet high in carbohydrates.

It is not clear what role carbohydrates play in weight gain. Carbohydrates increase blood glucose levels, which in effect induce pancreatic insulin release, and insulin stimulates fat tissue production and can cause weight gain. Most scientists believe that simple carbohydrates (sugars, fructose, desserts, soft drinks, alcohol, wine, etc.) contribute to weight gain because they are ingested more easily into the bloodstream than complex carbohydrates (pasta, brown rice, beans, potatoes, fresh fruits, etc.) and thus induce a more noticeable release of insulin during meals than complex carbohydrates. Some scientists believe that this higher release of insulin leads to weight gain.

5.Feeding frequency.

There is some debate about the relationship between feeding frequency (how often you eat) and weight. There are many studies that overweight people eat less often than normal-weight people. Scientists have observed that people who eat small meals four or five times a day have lower levels of cholesterol and lower and/or more healthy levels of blood sugar than people who eat less often (two or three large meals a day). One possible explanation is that small, regular meals yield steady levels of insulin, whereas large meals after meals cause large spikes in insulin.

6.Psychological factors.

Emotions impair eating habits for some individuals. In reaction to feelings such as depression, sorrow, pain, or frustration, often people eat excessively. While most overweight people have no more health symptoms than normal weight people, binge eating is problematic for about 30% of people seeking care for serious weight issues.

7.Disease.

Those related to obesity are conditions like hypothyroidism, insulin resistance, polycystic ovary syndrome, and Cushing's syndrome. Many disorders can lead to obesity, such as Prader-Willi syndrome.

8.Social issues:

Social issues are linked to obesity. Lack of money to purchase healthy food or lack of safe walking or fitness facilities will increase the risk of obesity.

What Happens When You Eat

Protein, fats, and starch are the main components in food. Protein is vital to the body's internal and cellular repair; protein is used in the cells for development and nutrition through excess fat accumulation, while carbohydrates are energy given foods. Carbohydrates are converted into glucose for energy in the bloodstream, and this is commonly referred to as "blood sugar." If sugar becomes excess in the system, it becomes toxic; thus, the pancreas releases insulin that brings the excess glucose into the liver and muscles to be processed as glycogen. Many of the foods we eat increase the development of insulin, and the remaining insulin starts to build up over a long period of time, allowing the body to build up an insulin resistance. There's weight gain at this stage, and that contributes to obesity.

An average person will store up to 15 grams of glycogen body weight per pound. The leftovers are processed as fat when there is excess glycogen in the blood. With the disorganized and disproportionate way people eat nowadays, the body waits around for glucose from foods which it then stores as fat for a fasting period that never comes. This leads to an imbalance in energy levels because carbohydrate is being consumed regularly rather than using the fat that has been stored in the body. Such a lifestyle leads to weight gain, obesity, and diabetes.

body. Such a lifestyle leads to weight gain, obesity, and diabetes.

What Happens When You Fast

Rather than use glucose when the body is fasting; it switches to fatty acids. This process happens when there is an increase in lipolysis (the breakdown of stored fat in your white adipose tissue into fatty acids and glycerol in the bloodstream). The free fatty acids are then used for energy, repair, and growth. In the event, they are not used; they are re-esterified as fat in your body.

The fatty acids in the bloodstream start to increase 12 hours after your last meal. This means that all body fat start to float around in the blood, waiting to be used. Within 24 hours of fasting, the amount of fatty acids reduces drastically in 72 hours the fatty acids peak and plateau. When fasting, the body releases twice the amount of fat into the bloodstream that is needed of the normal body function. People are always scared that they won't have the required energy to carry out their daily duties, but fasting actually makes the body oversaturated with fatty acids which makes the body have an excess amount of energy. Muscles and other tissues increase their ability to store fat when fasting; therefore, extra fatty acids may be stored there or used in different biosynthetic and metabolic pathways.

Fasting encourages the organs in the body to use and store fat. When fasting, the fat in the body no longer sits as a backup energy source; instead, it is being used by the body. This way of burning fat is called "fat-burning mode." During this period the body becomes super-efficient at processing fat which means tissues and other organs in the body use the fat for energy.

The Body's Reaction To Fasting

Here's what's happening to your body during a fasting period:

•Body fat breakdown

This is the part that contributes to weight loss and helps to reduce the risk of heart disease, strokes, obesity, diabetes, etc.

•Cholesterol deposits break down

Waste is removed easily through a fast–and this involves cholesterol, which is usually contained inside the blood vessel lining. The cholesterol levels may actually rise as the body detoxifies within the first week of the fast, but it will decrease.

•Mechanical fibrinolysis.

Dangerous blood clots can be broken down more easily while you're on a fast. This method is referred to as fibrinolysis.

•Speeding up autolysis.

Every cell in the body has its own destruction's seeds. If the need emerges, the cell can release and self-destruct its own self-destructive enzymes. It's autolysis. During the pace, the autolysis process leads to the breakdown of this type of tissue that has inhibited normal functioning.

•Lower diuresis.

Diuresis is the elimination of salt and water from the kidneys. The body naturally and automatically removes salt and water while fasting without destroying the tissues of the body. This diuresis is a tremendous benefit to wellbeing.

•The phagocytosis has intensified.

When fasting, the body's protective army of white blood cells is increasing its ability to destroy virulent bacteria and digest waste material. The fasting person's white blood cells were much more effective in killing virulent bacteria.

The Science Behind the Fast

Like any dietary plan that spreads over health and diet cultures rapidly, intermittent fasting has been suspected of being a fad but the evidence behind fasting's effectiveness is already clear— and increasing.

There are several hypotheses as to why intermittent fasting performs so well but stress has to do with the most widely studied — and most proven— benefit.

The term stress has been constantly vilified but some stress is actually beneficial to your health. Workout, for example, is actually a burden on the body (specifically on the muscles and cardiovascular system), but this particular stress ultimately makes the body healthier as long as you add the correct amount of recovery time into your exercise routine.

Intermittent fasting stresses the body in the same way that exercise does, according to Mark Mattson, who is the senior investigator for the National Institute on Aging. It puts the cells under mild stress when you deny the body food for a set period of time. Over time cells respond to that tension by learning how to better cope with it. If the body handles depression differently, it has an improved ability to resist illness.

Good Stress versus Bad Stress

While some kinds of stress are essential for the body to help it develop and evolve, there aren't other forms of stress. Distinguishing between "good" and "bad" stresses is crucial, so you can get a grip on the bad ones. A part of your brain called the amygdala recognizes that stress as a threat to your health when you're exposed to stress. In response to this threat, the amygdala sends a message for release of corticotrophin-releasing hormone, or CRH, to another part of your brain called the hypothalamus. CRH then activates another part of your brain to release adrenocorticotropic hormone, or ACTH, called the pituitary gland. ACTH release signals to the adrenal glands for the production and release of cortisol. The adrenal glands also release adrenaline which increases your blood pressure and heart rate. The production of cortisol helps to maintain proper blood pressure and fluid equilibrium, while briefly shutting down other body functions to conserve energy, such as digestion. In this scenario, once the imminent threat is gone, the levels of cortisol fall back down and normal body processes resumed.

Good stress, also referred to as eustress, is a moderate stress which most people regularly encounter. Instead of being harmful to the body, eustress encourages you to achieve a desired goal or result and is usually associated with some kind of satisfaction or anticipation when that goal is achieved. Types of eustress include preparing for an athletic event, working towards a timetable or exercising for a success to come. Research shows that in fact eustress can improve your brain function. The defining feature of eustress is that it's short-lived. Once the target has been achieved or the mission has been done, eustress goes away and the cortisol levels fall back and normalize, allowing the body time to recover.

Bad stress, or what is otherwise known as anxiety, is persistent, constant tension that hinders your productivity, or interferes with your everyday life. Instead of pushing you to accomplish your goals, distress makes achieving them more difficult. Distress induces elevated levels of cortisol and dopamine, which can contribute to impaired adrenal glands and normal hormonal signaling issues. Several persistent distress-related health problems include insomnia, heart disease, weight gain, and increased sensitivity to infections such as colds and flus. Types of depression include intimate toxic relationships, excessive stress at work and family loss or death.

Because everyone reacts differently to certain events, though, and has a different life experience, the distinction between good and bad stress can become fuzzy. The easiest way to determine if something is eustress or anxiety is to ask a few questions about yourself. Does that make you feel overwhelmed but still motivated? If so, then this is probably good pain. Does that make you feel stressed, exhausted and withdrawn? If so, then it's likely bad stress.

Fasting and "Bad" Stress

For most people, the discomfort that fasting imposes upon the body can be described as eustress. It's gentle and it offers health benefits that can drive you to get your ultimate goals running. However, if you're already in mental pain, you'll want to get that under control before you embed intermittent fasting into your routine. In the event of chronic stress, the body sends out cortisol constantly. If the cortisol levels remain elevated for an extended period of time, this may result in:

•Anxiety

•Depression

•Weight gain

•Headaches

•Problems with memory and concentration

•Difficulty sleeping

•Digestive issues

•Heart disease

With time, chronic stress often negatively affects the activity of your adrenal glands, which makes it more difficult for them to properly regulate hormones.

If you're already under a lot of chronic stress, it's extremely important to get your cortisol levels under control and your adrenal glands to work properly before you continue running hard. Through meditating, minimizing caffeine, getting enough sleep, eating a safe, healthy diet for a period of time before implementing fasting, and reducing physical exercise, you can and the cortisol levels. Meditative activities such as yoga can be effective for low-impact.

Getting Ready to Fast

Many forms of intermittent fasting entail some planning, excluding random fasting. Developing a schedule is one of the most important things you can do to prepare for your pace. What kind of intermittent fasting would you do? Which days and times are you going to fast? Which is the official start date for you? Creating a calendar for yourself and keeping it where you can see it all the time, is useful. You can even set timers to go off on your phone when it is time to start your fast and when it is time to start eating again. But you don't have to leap into a set schedule of fasting right away either: you should slowly ease yourself in to get the hang of it.

Easing Into Your Fast

If you're new to intermittent fasting or are used to having five or six small meals or regularly grazing throughout the day, jumping right into fasting can be a big transition. You don't have to make a complete change overnight; in fact if you slowly ease yourself into it, you may be more effective.

Begin with a change from five or six small meals throughout the day to three daily, scheduled meals. You don't have to feed within a certain time window anymore, just get your body used to the three meal plan routine and form. This will also require you throughout the day to eliminate snacking. Snacking is not banned when you're fasting intermittently, but when you're adapting it can be beneficial to avoid snacks during the start stages. You should add sweets during the day, as long as you eat them during your eating time, because your body gets used to fasting.

Once you've got the hang of a three meal routine, pick one meal to miss and stick to skipping it for a few weeks each day. Don't worry too much about which meal to skip; if it works better for you or your schedule, you can move meals later. The idea is to have your body used to going for an extended period of time without food. Sometimes the most difficult part of fasting is to prepare your mind to accept the idea of skipping meals, so this will get you used to that idea.

Once you've got the hang of skipping meals and you've decided which diet schedule you'll adopt, work your way up to the ultimate goal of fasting gradually. If you are going to follow the 16/8 method, for example, and you have decided that your eating window will fall between 11 a.m. And 7 p.m., when you normally eat breakfast at 7:30 a.m., continue by moving the breakfast back to 8:30 p.m. For a few days. So push it back another hour when you're used to the later breakfast and then another hour in a couple more days before your body's relaxed waiting until 11 a.m. Eating. Pushing back your feeding hours slowly will not only help ease you into the fast emotionally, it can also help prevent or reduce some of the initial physical effects that may arise during the early stages of intermittent fasting.

The next steps are to figure out what type of eating plan to follow and find some new and delicious recipes to incorporate into your plan. Fancy, complex meals are always tempting — and can be a great treat on the weekends— but it will be easier to keep things simple in the initial stages of your current fasting strategy. Choose recipes that are easy to prepare and made with ingredients that are readily available.

It is also good to scale back on your workout routine when you are just starting with intermittent fasting. You may be low on energy and enthusiasm at the very beginning stages of fasting. That is absolutely normal. Instead of going into any high-intensity drills, keep light on your workouts. Attempt the exercise, walk briskly or dive. When you usually do high-intensity training or a lot of strength training, cutting back that feel counterintuitive, but you can resume your workout routine within a few weeks after your body has adapted.

Chapter **2**

Types Of Intermittent Fasting

Another thing many people like about intermittent fasting is that it gives you plenty of options. As mentioned, you can do an irregular fast depending on your schedule and lifestyle in a few different ways. Some people find that during the week they have a couple of busy days, and so on those days they'll be fasting. Others like the idea of limiting their eating window every day and doing a small fast. The method you choose to quick is up to you. They can all be effective and will provide some of the benefits you're looking for. Let's take a look at some of the fasting options you can take with you, so you can choose the one you want.

Burn Fat And Slow Aging Through Metabolic Process Of Autophagy

Autophagy is a normal physiological process involving the purification of old or destroyed compounds within the body. Although it sounds a little nervous, the literal translation of autophagy is "self-eating." It comes from the Greek words autos, which translates to "self," and phagein, which means "eating." Christian de Duve, a Nobel Prize-winning physicist, coined the term autophagy after a group of researchers noticed an increase in lysosomes (the sections of the cells responsible for breaking down a scientist).

Autophagy plays a key role in preserving the body's homeostasis— a stable and healthy climate within itself. Your body constantly has defective or dying proteins and organelles (small, complex structures in each of the cells in your body). Such dead tissues, if allowed to accumulate in the body, may cause cell death, lead to reduced tissue and/or organ function and even become cancerous. During autophagy, the body marks damaged cell parts and unused body proteins. Such affected sections will be sent to the lysosomes, where they will be removed from the body. This process prevents harm from happening to them.

A board-certified radiation oncologist and associate professor at the University of Pittsburgh Medical Center, Dr. Colin

Champ explains this process as an unconscious recycling program. He believes that the autophagy cycle makes your body more effective by eliminating any defective parts, preventing any metabolic disease (such as obesity and diabetes), and avoiding cancerous (and potentially cancerous) growths.

There is also evidence that autophagy can help reduce chronic inflammation and improve natural immunity. Research shows that people unable to cause autophagy tend to carry more weight, sleep more often and have higher cholesterol levels and lower brain activity.

Fasting is one of the most powerful ways to stimulate autophagy in both the body and the brain, because the cycle is turned on by depriving the body of certain foods for a given period. As insulin goes up (after eating), glucagon (the hormone that functions counter to insulin) declines. Conversely, glucagon comes up as insulin goes down (after a time of nourishment). Glucagon increases when you fast, and activates autophagy.

Following a period of fasting, the amount of autophagosomes— the organelles responsible for removing the cellular waste — is significantly increasing in the body. Several studies have found that after fasting, the volume of autophagosomes will increase by as much as 300 percent.

While the science is clear that fasting increases autophagy, the one thing researchers do not agree on is exactly how to speed up the process to maximize it. It has been shown that each of the fasting methods stimulates autophagy, and no single method has proved better than another. Every approach has its own pros and cons so it is up to you eventually to determine which protocol works best for you.

The 16/8 Method

This is one of the most common methods in intermittent fasting that you can use. During this method you need to fast every day for about 14 to 16 hours, and eat the rest of the hours. You're still able to fit in two to three meals without a problem during this feeding period. This is more likely to fit into the meal routine you're used to, but it still controls you so you don't eat for the whole day.

This is simpler method than you think. It's as simple as not eating meals after dinner and then skipping breakfast or having a late breakfast at least. Okay, you're only fasting for 16 hours because you end your last meal at 8 at night and then eat nothing until noon the next day. Just be cautious about the late-night treats. When you eat them in the morning, you'll need to skip coffee.

Some people have problems with this because they feel hungry for breakfast in the morning and feel they need to eat. Simply move your breakfast to a bit later in the day. For example, if you choose to eat breakfast at 10 a.m. instead of eight, and then stop eating at 6 a.m., you'd still be within the 16-hour window.

As a woman it is advisable to go with this type of intermittent fasting. Women typically do better with these shorter fasts and it is advisable to go fasting for 14 and 15 hours, as this is more beneficial for you.

You are allowed to drink water, tea, coffee, and other non-caloric drinks during the fast to help reduce hunger pains. Furthermore, during your feeding time you should try to stick with healthier foods. During this time eating a lot of unhealthy food isn't a good idea. Most people like going on a low-carb diet when they're on sporadic fast because it helps with nausea and gives better outcomes.

The theory behind the 16/8 approach is focused on your circadian patterns and biological clock. According to Satchidananda Panda, a professor at the Salk Institute for Biological Studies and an expert in the field of biology and circadian rhythms, the body has not just one biological clock but several that make up the full circadian rhythm. There is one biological clock in your liver, one in your kidneys and one in your gut, and each of these clocks is switched on and turned off at different times, according to Panda.

The digestive system kicks into gear soon after you eat. Each organ involved in the digestive process turns on as food passes through your digestive tract, absorbs the food, and then turns off. When all digestive organs are turned off, the digestive system will have time to rest. It is during this period that the digestive system is doing its own "cleanup"— similar to a self-cleaning oven idea. All the remaining traces of food are cleaned out and the body is ready to start anew.

And, if you constantly put food in your mouth, your digestive system will never shut down, so it will never have enough time to perform its self-cleaning, which will have a negative impact on both your metabolism and overall health. Panda found through his study that giving the body an eight to twelve-hour window without food is best for your health. He says implementing a routine fasting period will help you lose weight (or maintain a heathy weight) and help stave off diabetes, high cholesterol, and obesity.

The Importance of Your Circadian Rhythm

It is helpful to know what your circadian rhythm is, and how it affects your body, to fully understand Panda's research. Often called a body clock or a biological clock, the circadian rhythm is a twenty-four-hour cycle that controls many of the physiological processes in your body, such as sleep and digestion. Your body receives signs about when to go to sleep, when to wake up and when to eat from your circadian rhythm.

Your circadian rhythm is internally controlled by a brain area called the hypothalamus, but it is largely affected by external, environmental indications such as temperature and light. For example, when it's dark outside, your eyes send a signal to your hypothalamus that it's time to sleep; your hypothalamus sends a message to the pineal gland (in another brain area) that activates melatonin (a hormone that helps you sleep), and you get sleepy. The opposite happens when it's light-out. Your eyes send out a signal to your hypothalamus, sending a signal to your pineal gland to reduce melatonin production. A dip in melatonin makes you get up and get ready for the day.

The 5:2 diet

Another viable option is the 5:2 diet. This fast tells you to eat normally during the week for five days, and to limit yourself to no more than 600 calories for each of the other two days. This is also sometimes referred to as the Fast Diet.

It is advised that women should eat about 500 calories on these fasting days. For example, you'll eat normally every day of the week and on Monday and Thursdays you'll consume only two small meals with a minimum of 500 calories. So long as you don't have them back to back, you can choose any day of the week as your fasting days. Choose your two busiest days of the week, and make those your days of fasting.

There aren't many reports out there about the 5:2 diet, but as it's intermittent fast, it will provide most of the benefits you're finding. You can get things done without having to worry about making meals all day.

Eat-Stop-Eat diet

The Eat-Stop-Eat diet allows you to avoid eating once or twice a week for 24 hours. This technique was first popularized by Brad Pilon and for some time has been a popular way of doing the intermittent fast. This fast can be done while still getting one meal a day. Every day, most people will have dinner and then eat nothing until the next day's supper. In the 24-hour abstinence cycle, that helps you to never go a full day without feeding but still crash.

However you like you should change this. When moving from breakfast to breakfast or lunch to lunch is better for you then you can choose one of those choices. You are permitted to have caffeine, tea, and other non-caloric liquids during your fast, to keep you hydrated, but you are not allowed to have any food at all.

Recall for one or two days a week you're just fasting. If eating regularly is the moment, you need to consume the same amount of food you'd have if you weren't on a fast. This will help you lose weight without doing any damage to your body.

The only problem with going on this kind of sporadic fast is that it is hard for most people to run for 24 hours. You should ease that into it, however. You may find that beginning with a shorter pace, such as the fast of 16 hours, will yield some good results and then continue fasting for longer periods of time. It can be difficult to go a whole day without food and most people tend to go with one of the other fasting choices to see the same results.

Alternate day fasting

With this option, you will go on a fast every alternate days. There are a few things you can take with you, and it depends on what appeals to your needs. Some of those fasts on your fasting days would cause you to have around 500 calories. You will note that most of the intermittent fasting laboratory studies used some variant of the easy alternate day to help determine all the health benefits. To most people it can be daunting for fast every other day.

Fasting every other day is definitely something you'll need to build up to. Forcing yourself to eat on alternate days can be a challenge. On this fasting schedule you'll probably feel very hungry many days a week, and it's hard to stick to over the long run.

Warrior Diet

This is another popular option for intermittent fasting that you can choose from. During the day, it involves eating small amounts of raw fruits and vegetables followed by a large meal at night. It requires you to walk the whole day, eat just enough to keep you happy and then feast within a four-hour feeding window at night. One of the first diets to include a sort of intermittent fasting is the Warrior diet.

Also included in the warrior diet are food choices which resemble the Paleo diet. Not only will you fast during most of the day and night celebrations, but you'll eat a diet full of unprocessed foods that sound like what you can see out in nature.

Spontaneous Meal Skipping

If you want to brace your body for intermittent fasting or you don't want to spend much time thinking about when you can feed, you should do this. With this fast, you don't have to think about implementing one of the intermittent fasting plans which are more formal. Occasionally, you'll probably miss any meals. You can do this if you're not hungry or if you're too tired for a meal. It's a big myth that to stop hunger, you have to eat food every few hours.

The liver is well prepared for enduring long periods without feeding. Missing out on a few meals is not detrimental to your health, particularly if you are not hungry or too busy.

You are technically fasting whenever you end up skipping a meal, or two. If you're too distracted on the way out of the door to get a snack just make sure you're eating a healthy lunch and dinner. If you're running out of errands and can't find a place to eat, so skipping out on a lunch is perfect. It won't cause any harm and really will help save you money.

Similar to some of the other choices, you probably won't see results as nice but it's better than nothing and it's a lot easier to work with. Perhaps try skipping a meal or two over the week or avoiding any meals when it's going for you.

As you can see, when you're ready to go on the sporadic quick, there are several different options you can deal with. Some of these will be simpler than others, and some will be better suited to your timetable. You will need to choose which quick is easiest for you to work in your everyday life.

Extended Fasting

While extended fasting belongs to a class of its own, understanding the difference between it and the other forms of intermittent fasting is significant. Extended fasting is any form of fast which lasts longer than 24 hours. Lengthy fasting can often last a week and many of these lengthy fasts require simply drinking liquids.

Throughout medical and surgical settings, these types of fasts are more normal and are usually done when the body needs to experience substantial recovery or when the ability to feed is impaired. You should not continue a sustained fast without a medical professional's advice and supervision.

Other Ways to Increase Autophagy

While fasting is the most powerful way to stimulate autophagy, by exercising and maintaining a ketogenic diet you can kick on this cycle as well. That's why many people who decide to fast also follow a ketogenic diet: it's a double whammy for cellular cleansing. The ketogenic diet helps promote autophagy by tricking the body into thinking it's going without food, so you can see the same improvements in metabolism. If you drastically lower sugars, the body is forced to turn instead to use fat as an energy source. Doing this also holds low levels of insulin and high levels of glucagon— a must for starting autophagy.

Exercise is another powerful way to stimulate autophagy and it has been shown that regular exercise kills cancer cells because of this. One study published in Autophagy showed that after jogging on a treadmill for thirty minutes, autophagy increases significantly and continues to increase to eighty total minutes

of exercise when it appears to level out. For intensive exercise
the result is seen to a greater degree.

Best Types Of Intermittent Fasting For Women

There is no one-size-fits-all approach when it comes to diet. This also applies to fasting intermittently.

In general terms, women should take fasting in a more relaxed way than men.

This could include shorter periods of fasting, fewer days of fasting and/or eating a limited amount of calories on the days of fasting.

Here are some of the best forms of female intermittent fasting:

- Crescendo Method: Fasting on two or three days a week for 12–16 hours. Fasting days should be non-consecutive and evenly spaced throughout the week (e.g. Tuesday, Wednesday, and Friday).

- Eat-stop-eat (also known as the 24-hour protocol): 24-hour full fast once or twice a week (for women, at most two days a week). Begin with fasts of 14–16 hours, and build up slowly.

- 5:2 Diet (also known as "The Fast Diet"): Limit calories to 25 percent of your usual intake (about 500 calories) for

two days a week and eat the other five days "normally."
Space for one day between days of fasting.

•Modified Alternate-Day Fasting: Fasting on non-fasting days every other day but eating "normally." On a fasting day, you are allowed to consume 20–25 percent of your daily calorie intake (around 500 calories).

•Method 16/8 (also known as the "Leangains Method"): Run for 16 hours a day and eat all the calories within an eight-hour window. It is advised that women start with 14-hour fasts, and eventually build up to 16 hours.

Whatever you choose, well eating during the non-fasting periods is still important. If during the non-fasting periods you eat a large amount of unhealthy, calorie dense foods, you may not experience the same weight loss and health benefits.

The best approach at the end of the day is one that you can handle and maintain over the long term, and that does not result in any negative health consequences.

Why Should I Try Intermittent Fasting?

There are many different diet plans you can choose from. Some help limit your intake of carb and focus on the good fats and proteins. Some will limit the fat intake and concentrate on healthy and good carbohydrates.

With all of the market choices, and with at least a couple of them being real weight loss options, you may be confused as to why you should go with intermittent fasting. Each section looks at the different benefits of intermittent fasting and how it will make a difference for your wellbeing.

1.Changes the function of hormones, genes, and cells

Several things happen to your body, if you don't eat for a while. For starters, the body will start cell repair processes and will change some of the hormone levels, which will make it easier to access accumulated body fat. Some improvements that may arise in the body include:

- Insulin levels: the insulin levels may decrease slightly, making consuming fat harder for the stomach.

- Human growth hormone: growth hormone blood levels will rise sharply. Higher levels of this hormone can help muscle build up and fat burn.

•Cellular repair: The body starts essential mechanisms of cellular repair, such as eliminating the waste from the cells.

•Gene expression: There are some positive improvements in several genes that will help you live longer and shield yourself from illness.

2.Lose weight and body fat

Most people are going on an irregular ride for weight loss. Intermittent fasting in most cases will of course help you eat fewer meals. You'll end up taking fewer calories, resulting in a weight loss.

Fasting also boosts hormone function to facilitate weight loss. Higher levels of growth hormones and lower insulin are helping the body break down fat and use it for energy. That's why short-term fasting can increase your metabolism by three percent or more.

It increases your metabolic rate on the one hand, so that you burn more calories while also reducing how much you eat. People have been able to lose up to 8 per cent of their body weight in less than 24 hours, according to a 2014 study of scientific research on intermittent fasting.

3.Helps with diabetes

Type 2 diabetes is a condition which has become common over the last few decades. Anything that reduces your tolerance to insulin will help lower your level of blood sugar and protect you against type 2 diabetes. Several studies show how intermittent fasting in insulin resistance can benefit and can help bring about a dramatic reduction of blood sugar levels.

Blood sugar was reduced by three to six percent in several intermittent fasting trials, while insulin was reduced by twenty to thirty-one percent. One research on diabetic rats also found that intermittent fasting could shield the rat from kidney damage, a frequent problem with more severe forms of diabetes. It indicates that for anyone with a higher risk of developing type 2 diabetes intermittent fasting may be a good option.

One study which showed that blood sugar control could actually get worse for women after a few weeks of going on the intermittent hard. It is advised that you speak with your doctor before you initiate some sort of diet plan.

4.Simplifies life

Although this may not be considered a health advantage like the others, noting this is still a significant one. Some people find intermittent fasting will improve their lives. They find that they don't need to focus too much on the calories they consume, as long as they stay within the hours that they can feed. They can go a couple of days a week without worrying about making a dinner. Ultimately, the diet plan will make life easier for you.

You will end up with less stress in your life if you can take out some of the tasks you need to do during the day and concentrate on something else. We all know how much stress will affect our health and life adversely. If you can reduce stress, being the healthiest version of yourself is much easier.

5.Good for the heart

Heart disease is considered as one of the world's greatest killers. Intermittent fasting can assist with some of these risk factors, such as lower blood sugar rates, inflammatory markers, triglycerides in the blood, cholesterol and blood pressure.

The biggest problem is that there have been a lot of studies on intermittent fasting on wildlife. They need more research to check intermittent fasting and human heart safety.

6.Can help with cancer

Every year lots of women die from cancer. This terrible illness is marked by unchecked cell growth. Fasting has been shown to have some significant advantages when it comes to your metabolism which could lead to lower cancer risk.

Several human studies indicate that people with cancer that fasted may have been able to reduce some of the side effects that come with chemotherapy.

7.Good for the brain

Intermittent fasting can help to improve metabolic features which are also known to help the brain stay healthy. This might include dealing with insulin resistance, raising blood sugar levels, lowering inflammation and oxidative stress.

Several experiments on rats have been performed that demonstrate how intermittent fasting can help to increase the growth of new nerve cells, thereby increasing the function of the brain. Fasting may also help to increase levels of the neurotrophic factor derived from the brain. It can cause depression as well as some other brain problems when the brain is defective in that.

8.Helps with cellular repair

When we go on a quick, a waste removal process known as autophagy can be triggered by the cells within the body. It involves breaking down the cells and metabolizing the proteins that can no longer be used. It could help protect the body from illnesses such as Alzheimer's and cancer, with an increased amount of autophagy.

9.May prevent Alzheimer's

Alzheimer's is among the most common neurodegenerative diseases. There is no treatment for Alzheimer's, but stopping it from happening is your best course of action. One study done on rats found that intermittent fasting could delay the onset of Alzheimer's disease, or at least reduce its severity.

Several case reports have shown that a change in lifestyle that included some regular, or at least frequent, short-term fasts has helped improve Alzheimer's symptoms in 9 out of 10 cases. Animal studies also show that this kind of fasting will help protect against other neurodegenerative diseases, such as Huntington's and Parkinson's disease.

Although most of these experiments have been conducted on primates, the results appear positive. Intermittent fasting is a phenomenon and relatively new are findings in how it makes the body safer. Studying all of the benefits of intermittent fasting will take some time.

10.Intermittent fasting could help you to live longer

One of intermittent fasting's most exciting things is that it can help you live longer. Several rat studies have shown how intermittent fasting can help prolong their lifetime-similar to what happens when you go on a continuous restriction on calories. The results had been drastic in some of the trials. When the rats fasted every other day, they ended up living 83 per cent longer in one of them than the rats who did not fast.

While confirming an improvement in longevity has been difficult as intermittent fasting has yet to be tested on people long enough to prove that, it is still a popular idea for those who try to prevent ageing. Given that metabolism with this diet has established effects, it's no wonder that people assume that intermittent fasting will help them live longer and healthier lives.

As you can see, the intermittent fasting diet has many advantages to go with. We've only touched on a few of them, but a number of research have been conducted about the consequences of this diet and why it can help you. Whether you're trying to improve the health of your brain, live longer, lose weight or get more strength, intermittent fasting will make your life better.

Health Benefits Of Intermittent Fasting For Women

Not only does intermittent fasting help your waistline, it can also reduce your risk of contracting a variety of chronic diseases.

•Heart Health

Heart disease is the world's number one cause of death. High blood pressure, high LDL cholesterol and high concentrations of triglycerides are among the main risk factors for heart disease growth.

One test of 16 obese men and women has shown intermittent fasting in just eight weeks to lower blood pressure by 6 percent. It was also observed in the same study that intermittent fasting decreased LDL cholesterol by 25% and triglycerides by 32%

The evidence for the correlation between intermittent fasting and increased levels of LDL cholesterol and triglyceride is not conclusive though. A research of 40 normal-weight individuals showed that four weeks of intermittent fasting during Ramadan's Islamic holiday did not lead to a reduction in LDL cholesterol or triglycerides.

Higher-quality trials with more rigorous approaches are required before researchers can better understand the effects on heart health of intermittent fasting.

•Diabetes

Intermittent fasting can also help you effectively manage and reduce the diabetes risk. Compared to prolonged calorie restriction, intermittent fasting tends to mitigate some of the diabetes risk factors.

This is done primarily by increasing insulin levels and raising exposure to insulin. Six months of intermittent fasting decreased insulin levels by 29 percent and insulin resistance by 19 percent in a randomized controlled trial of more than 100 overweight or obese people. The levels of blood sugar remained the same.

Moreover, in individuals with pre-diabetes, 8–12 weeks of intermittent fasting have been shown to lower insulin levels by 20–31 percent and blood sugar levels by 3–6 percent, a condition in which blood sugar levels are elevated but not high enough for diagnosis.

Intermittent fasting, however, may not be as beneficial in terms of blood sugar for women as it is for men. A small study found that control of blood sugar worsened for women after 22 days of alternate-day fasting, while no adverse effect on men's blood sugar was seen.

Despite this side effect, a reduction in insulin and insulin resistance would likely still reduce the risk of diabetes, especially for pre-diabetes individuals.

•Weight Loss

If done properly, intermittent fasting can be a simple and effective way to lose weight, because regular short-term fasts can help you consume fewer calories and shed pounds.

For short-term weight loss, several studies suggest that intermittent fasting is as effective as traditional calorie-restricted diets.

A 2018 study of overweight adult studies found intermittent fasting resulted in a 15 lbs (6.8 kg) average weight loss over 3–12 months.

One study found intermittent fasting in overweight or obese adults over a span of 3–24 weeks decreased body weight by 3–8 per cent. The study also showed that participants over the same time lowered their waist circumference by 3–7 per cent.

It should be remembered that the long-term effects of intermittent fasting on women's weight loss continue to be seen.

Intermittent fasting tends to help in weight loss in the short term. The amount you lose, though, will probably depend on how many calories you eat during non-fasting hours and how long you stick to the diet.

- It May Help You Eat Less

Switching to extended fasting will help you eat less, obviously.

One study found that when their food intake was limited to a four-hour window, young men ate 650 fewer calories per day.

Another research in 24 healthy men and women investigated the impact on eating habits of a long, 36-hour fast. Given the post-fast day intake of extra calories, participants reduced their total calorie level by 1,900 calories, which is a significant reduction.

Other Health Benefits

A number of studies on humans and animals indicate that intermittent fasting could also offer other health benefits.

- Reduced inflammation: Several studies show intermittent fasting can reduce main inflammatory markers. Chronic inflammation may give rise to weight gain and various health problems.

- Psychological well-being improved: One study found that eight weeks of intermittent fasting reduced depression and binge eating behaviors while improving body image in obese adults.

- •Increased longevity: intermittent fasting was shown to extend lifetime by 33–83 percent in rats and mice. The implications on human lifespan are yet to be known.

- •Preserve muscle mass: it suggests that intermittent fasting is more effective in maintaining muscle mass compared to constant calorie restriction. Even at rest, greater muscle mass makes you burn more calories.

Specifically, the health benefits of intermittent fasting for women in well-designed human studies need to be investigated more thoroughly before any conclusions can be drawn.

What To Expect

As with any change in lifestyle, intermittent fasting can at first be difficult. You can experience a drop of motivation or some irritability. You may feel very hungry and struggle to stick to your diet. Or you might feel great right off the bat, immediately experience positive results and feel energized and motivated by your new lifestyle. This depends on your body. There are, however, some things that are likely to happen when you adapt to your new routine. When you know what to expect and have some tools ready to handle any challenges that may arise, your chances of long-term success are far greater.

How Your Mind Will Feel

There's a famous quote saying, "Your subconscious is going to quit a thousand times before your body is going to," and another quote that says, "Your body can take virtually anything. The general message behind these two important quotations is that often, when you give up, it's not because you have hit your physical limit, it's because you've exceeded your emotional limit. In other words, your ego is reminding you that when it really does, your body can not withstand a task physically.

The Negativity Bias

The brain has a propensity to be more reactive to negative things than to positive things. This phenomenon is called the tendency of negativity — and it can be extremely potent. The evolutionary function of the negativity bias is to shield you from possible threats, but in modern times, threats such as those encountered by your ancestors are rapidly diminishing. As a result, this negativity bias is not needed as often, because it is not as helpful as it once was. In fact, this bias makes it more difficult for you to be present and calm, as you are always on the alert and anticipating a negative event rather than appreciating the moment. The good news is that you can potentially retrain your brain so it doesn't get too easily back into the negativity bias.

The Power of Positive Thinking

Positive thinking and assumptions are not just phenomena of the New Age: they are powerful tools that can potentially rewire the brain's neurons— a phenomenon known as neuroplasticity. If you indulge in positive thinking daily and say positive affirmations, it makes it easier for your brain to respond more positively to issues, rather than resorting to its normal negative bias automatically. And the more you work, the better it is to think positively for your personality.

Your subconscious mind can fight the transition when you continue with intermittent fasting and will do all it can to get you back to your old routine. Once you know that, negative thought patterns and unconstructive self-talk are harder to become mindful of. You may find yourself thinking stuff like, "This is way too hard," "I'm hungry," or "I won't hurt a little snack outside my fasting window." Those feelings are all signs that the show is running the negativity bias. If your head tries to convince you it's too hard, realize that communicating is this stigma and react by saying something like, "I'm stronger than my emotions. I will accomplish my goals, and will reach them.

While performing positive affirmations daily and adjusting your negative self-talk, you can also shut down your negativity bias by reflecting on the bigger picture. Find the main reasons to fast. Is it weight loss? Gaining more strength and emotional clarity? Does your blood sugar balance? Does your brain sustain healthy? Whatever the motives are, write them down on a piece of paper or sticky notes and put them somewhere you will often see them, like in the fridge. Read the notes and remember your main goals and why you started in the first place when you feel these negative thoughts start creeping in. This can help you see the bigger picture along the way, which will get you through any small speed bumps.

Once you have gone past the initial stages of intermittent fasting, you'll probably notice any major changes. Not only will your negative self-talk and aversion to cynicism diminish, but you will also have greater clarity of mind. Intermittent fasting helps to heighten brain fog and promote focus. You can find that simple tasks are harder, and you can concentrate more on your job. You may also feel less of a "monkey mind"—intrusive, fast thinking that distracts you from the task at hand and interferes with your productivity. You may note changes in your efficiency and energy levels. Your memories may feel better and it may become harder to remember new information than it used to be. In your moods and attitudes, you might also note a stabilization— even less tension and a more cheerful disposition.

How Your Body Will Feel

It's impossible to say precisely how the body would react during the initial stages of intermittent fasting, because everyone is different and you may respond differently than someone else. Nonetheless, after beginning intermittent fasting, there are a few issues generally happening in most individuals. If you're used to eating 5 or 6 times a day, you may feel these symptoms to a greater extent than if you're only consuming 3 meals a day with little snacking.

It's normal to feel intensified hunger and cravings as the body adjusts to intermittent fasting. This is often more a mental or emotional hunger than actual hunger. There may also be fatigue, low energy and irritability. Upon standing it can feel a little dizzy, weak, or light-headed. The severity of these effects can differ based on several factors, including your past eating habits, but they should not be overly disruptive and should decline within a week or so.

Your blood sugar and insulin levels start to stabilize after the initial adjustment period, and you'll begin to reap the benefits of intermittent fasting. One of the first things you'll possibly find is heightened passion. Throughout the day you may experience a sustained energy, instead of feeling up and successful in the morning but then being struck with the dreaded afternoon depression about two or three p.m., you may feel constant energy. This is because your blood sugar doesn't spike and drop like it does when you eat multiple meals all day long.

Inflammation may also decrease, so any puffiness in your hair, head, hands, or feet can continue to decrease. Chronic aches and pains that have become a regular part of your day that lessen or go away altogether. Then you might begin to notice that you're losing a few extra pounds, falling asleep quicker, and improving the quality of your sleep. You're going to toss and turn less at night and as a result you're going to wake up feeling refreshed and relaxed rather than groggy and disorientated. You may also find it easier to get through your exercises if you exercise regularly.

A good way to keep track of changes is to write down any symptoms you may feel before your intermittent fasting plan starts. Try digging hard and be really thorough, including listing things that you've been grappling with for a long time or that you believe your eating habits have nothing to do with it. Go back and rewrite your list after you've been fasting for a couple of weeks and compare the two lists. Afterwards, revise the list every few weeks. This can help you track changes you might not even anticipate and you'll actually be pleasantly surprised.

Staving Off Hunger

You'll feel hungry in the initial stages of intermittent fasting — there's no way around that. Fortunately, you can stave off both physical and mental hunger without breaking your fast with a knowledge of hunger signals and a few simple techniques.

The Psychology of Hunger

Hunger is tricky because there is real, physiological hunger, on the one hand; mental hunger, on the other. Simply put: when the stomach is hollow real hunger exists. You can feel your stomach's physical emptiness along with a weakness or a dip in energy. Psychological hunger is the result of a desire to eat out of habit or boredom, or outward indications. While you may do these things subconsciously, you can alter how they affect you when you become aware of them. Instead of behaving carelessly because you're starving at a social event, with your significant other, pay attention to how you really feel. Are you really hungry, or are you just being tempted by one of those indications? If it's the latter, you can either adjust your environment or use one of a few helpful strategies to curb your hunger.

Sensory Cues

As the name implies, anything that stimulates your desire to eat by stimulating your senses is an external sensory signal. You might smell your favorite meal, for example, or see a jar full of freshly baked cookies. You can even read a description of a meal in a magazine, or watch a TV cooking show, and start feeling hungry, even if you're not physically hungry. Exposure to external sensory signals will significantly increase the desire to eat, even if your stomach is full and you're not very hungry, according to the study.

Social Cues

Although food is meant to be a source of sustenance, it has become a way to entertain people and others. Going out to eat at a restaurant is now a favorite pastime, and you can never go to a party or other gathering without seeing all kinds of food available. In many of these instances, even if you're not thirsty, you certainly should eat; sometimes you won't even know it. For one study, published in the American Journal of Health Practice, the students were told to eat alone and then advised to eat with others to investigate the impact of social cues on food consumption. We drank 60 per cent more calories when these students ate with others than when we ate alone. Another research, published in the Consumer Research Journal, has shown that dining with a romantic partner can also affect the amount of food you eat. When one participant ate more in the test, the other presumably should eat more too.

Normative Cues

Normative signs are things that affect the amount of food you consume, such as portion size or plate size. You may not even understand that these things affect you, but research shows that you appear to feed yourself better when you use bigger dishes, and as a result eat more.

Drink Up (Water, That Is)

Water should be your best friend during your times of fasting (and in general). You have probably heard that dehydration is often mistaken for hunger, and remaining hydrated will help to reduce any false symptoms of hunger. Just waking up and drinking 8 ounces of water. When you go to sleep you should relax by having a glass of water at your nightstand. Drink water daily throughout the day and have at least half of your body weight ingested in ounces every day. If you are doing a lot of exercise or otherwise wasting water, you may need to drink even more than that. For every cup of coffee or other diuretic you drink, you will also need to add an extra glass of water so keep that in mind. The more hydrated you are, the less likely you can come across false signals of hunger.

Buying a reusable water bottle which you really love might be helpful. It might sound stupid, but sometimes foods actually taste better when you drink them from certain glasses. There are many firms out there that make bottles of stainless steel, insulated water that keep your water cold for hours. Whenever necessary, you can refill these water bottles and bring them wherever you go so you'll always have clean water at hand. Use of a reusable water bottle as an added bonus is also better for the environment.

Stay Busy

How many times did you think you were starving but it turned out you just felt bored? You're waiting around watching TV for one minute and scouring through the pantry for something to snack on the next. Then a whole bag of chips is gone before you know it and you don't even know how that happened.

The best way to avoid this thoughtless snacking is to keep yourself–and your hands–busy. Fill the time with entertainment and friends. Perform creative projects or completely immerse yourself in the work. Call a friend or go for a walk around the neighborhood if you feel boredom creeping in and are tempted to eat just for the sake of eating.

Look for (and Eliminate) Triggers

Look for stuff that causes your internal hunger— and then stop it. You may have been on autopilot up until now when it comes to eating. You haven't really paid attention to what's happening around you or what's affecting the quantity or types of food that you consume. Do you have one significant other, for starters, that drinks half as much as you do? Should you keep your favorite snacks within reach in the pantry or refrigerator any time you open the doors? Should you schedule social events around food? What types of restaurants do you choose for these events, or what types of dishes do you and your friends make?

Figuring out that will encourage you to eat more— or choose unhealthy foods — will go a long way not only to sustain intermittent fasting as a habit, but also to protect your safety. Surround yourself with people who embrace changes in your lifestyle and keep away from people who might hinder your efforts, or restrict time with them.

Reduce Stress Levels

Stress is a major issue around the world. Approximately 77 percent of women in the U.S. report consistently experiencing stress-induced physical symptoms and 33 percent of those people say they are coping with extreme stress. Stress may result in weight gain, as well as heart disease, diabetes, fatigue, insomnia, anxiety, and gastrointestinal issues.

One of the immediate ways in which tension leads to weight gain is by enticing you to reach for convenient items such as pizza or ice cream that you may not be afraid of when the stress levels are more under check. Even though some people tend to lose their appetite under high stress, many have an increased appetite for food that is not conducive to a healthy lifestyle.

Whatever type of stress-eating you fall under, you'll want to find ways to manage the pain. However, when you fall into the latter category, stress management is particularly helpful in keeping hunger signals at bay. When your stress levels are under control, you'll be able to focus on your eating plan and take steps to help you achieve your goals.

Sleep

The value of sleep cannot be overestimated— not only to stay away from malnutrition, but to the overall health. Sleep is nourishing so restorative, and if you don't get enough of it, it can throw you off in all ways entirely. It's easy to skimp on sleeping when you're stressed out in favor of trying to knock a few more things off your to - do list but don't! Bed time is when rebuilding and recharging your brain and body, and controlling your stress levels and appetite hormones is important. Rest often leads to increased levels of attitude and vitality, ability to focus, and willpower — which is particularly important in the early stages of intermittent fasting.

There are two main hormones involved in the hunger response-ghrelin and leptin. Ghrelin is the hormone of appetite, and when released into your bloodstream it tells the brain, "Yeah, you're hungry; let's feed." Leptin is the hormone of satiation, and it says, "Alright, you're full now. You should stop eating. "The amount of ghrelin the body produces increases when you are sleep-deprived, while the amount of leptin it produces decreases. As a consequence, the body tells you regularly that you're starving and rarely, if ever, telling you you're full. Besides this hormonal imbalance, when you are sleep-deprived your metabolism slows down, so you don't cook off the food you eat as quickly.

Always make sleep a priority. Make sure that you hit the sheets after 10 p.m. And get seven to nine hours of disturbed sleep every night. Just like with the intermittent fasting strategy, even on holidays, try to stick to the same sleep schedule (the same bedtime and wake-up time). It helps to regulate the circadian rhythm as does fasting. Make sure that your room is dark and free of unnecessary noise or lights, particularly from electronic devices. Keep your phone in another room or turn it off so your sleep won't be disrupted by any alerts. Place all the appliances away at least an hour before bedtime. Watch the consumption of caffeine and after two pm turn to decaffeinated beverages.

Be patient with yourself and give it time; it's not going to be easy to change your eating and sleeping patterns right away, but if you give it all, as time goes on it will become much easier.

Safety and Side Effects

Modified forms of intermittent fasting appear safe to most women.

That said, some studies have documented several side effects on fasting days including nausea, mood swings, lack of concentration, lost strength, headaches and bad breath.

There are also some news stories of women who report having interrupted their menstrual cycle while following an intermittent fasting diet.

If you have a medical condition, consult your doctor before attempting intermittent fasting.

Medical consultation is particularly important for women who:

•Have a history of eating disorders.

•Have diabetes or regularly experience low blood sugar levels.

•Are underweight, malnourished or have nutritional deficiencies.

•Are pregnant, breastfeeding or trying to conceive.

•Have fertility problems or a history of amenorrhea (missed periods).

Intermittent fasting is starting to have a good safety profile at the end of the day. Yet if you encounter any issues — such menstrual cycle loss — stop immediately.

Effects Of Intermittent Fasting On Women

Many evidence suggests that intermittent fasting may not be as helpful to some women as it is to men.

One study showed that regulation of blood sugar significantly decreased in women after three weeks of intermittent fasting, which wasn't the case in men.

There are also many anecdotal stories of women who, after beginning intermittent fasting, have undergone improvements to their menstrual cycles.

These changes arise as women's bodies are extremely sensitive to restricting calories.

If calorie intake is low — such as fasting for too long or too often— a small part of the brain is affected, called the hypothalamus.

This may interfere with the secretion of gonadotropin-releasing hormone (GnRH), which helps release two reproductive hormones: luteinizing hormone (LH) and follicle-stimulating hormone (FSH).

You run the risk of irregular periods, infertility, poor bone health and other health effects when these hormones cannot communicate with the ovaries.

Although there are no corresponding human studies, rat experiments have shown that 3–6 months of alternate-day fasting in female rats caused a decrease in ovarian size and erratic menstrual cycles.

For these reasons women should find a relaxed solution to intermittent fasting, such as shorter periods of fasting and fewer days of fasting.

Tips And Tools To Stay Focused

The most important thing that you can do is to have a plan to ensure your success with intermittent fasting. The first step is to decide what sort of fasting you'll do. Once that method of fasting has been decided, make a timetable. Can you fast every day? Which times are you going to fly, and what times are you going to be feeding? After you've established a schedule, another critical component will decide what you'll eat when it's time to get into your fed. Should you follow a specific dietary routine (such as the ketogenic diet or Paleo diet) or will you adhere to a simple clean-eating schedule without any particular "rules"?

1.Incorporate Meal Prep

Getting the basics down, planning your meals will help keep you on track and prevent you from getting into temptation for an unhealthy meal. Research shows that people who prepare their meals in advance experience greater success in their health and nutrition plans as well as long-term gains in time and money. You will make adjustments to your menus and your prepping schedule as you follow the rhythm of intermittent fasting and a new way of life.

Meal-Prepping Tips

One of the most important components of good meal preparation is getting organized. It may seem difficult to sit down and arrange meals and type everything out, or like a waste of time, but it will eventually save you hours down the road.

The amount of food that you make in advance and the amount of time you spend preparing is solely your responsibility. Many people spend three to four hours prepping meals on Sunday for the whole week. Many spend a few hours on Sunday preparing meals for the next few days, and then spend a couple more hours on Wednesday preparing meals for the remainder of the week. Whatever type of meal you select, organizing is important.

2.Figure Out Your Plan

You'll need to build your meal plan first. You should schedule a couple of days, a week or even the whole month. Find simple recipes, then write down what you're going to eat and when. The excitement may tempt you to look for fancy, new recipes or a lot of variety when you start with intermittent fasting and meal planning, but when you're in the initial stages of a new lifestyle change, one of the most beneficial things you can do is stick to the basics and not overcomplicate things.

Stick to foods you're already familiar with and recipes that won't take too long to prepare or require you to learn new cooking skills or purchase new cooking tools. After you get used to the basics and adjust your body and mind to the changes, there is plenty of time for you to try new things. The point of prepping your meal is to make you feel less stressed, and not add unnecessary tension.

There are online menu plans and trackers, as well as phone apps that you can use to keep track of your meals, but if automation is not your thing, you don't need any advanced gadgets or devices. Recording everything in a journal will keep it simple.

3.Write Your Grocery List

Once you've got your recipes together and written out your meal plan, it's time to figure out what you need. Before you write your grocery list, check your refrigerator and pantry so you don't buy things you already have. After compiling a list of things you've got on hand, write a list of the remaining items you'll need to complete your weekly recipes and meals (or for whatever length of time you've selected).

Through arranging your list of groceries based on where products are sold in the store you can save even more time. You can list all the meats together; together you can manufacture all the items and all the refrigerated items. For any deals or specialty items, organize your lists by store, if you need to go to different stores.

4.Make Your Meals

A great way to save money is to go shopping the same day you'll be preparing your meals. This way, when you get home, you won't have to put away as many food items— you can jump right into preparing your meals. Divide them into separate containers by portion size until the meals are prepared, and name them accordingly. So when you're ready to eat you're going to have a lunch ready to go and if you're bringing a food with you on the go it's going to be easy to bring.

5.Take Pictures and Measurements

If weight loss is one of your targets, don't rely on the scale alone. Your actual weight will fluctuate significantly from day to day, and even when your body is going through a huge transition, you might not see big changes in the figures. You can use the scale as a tool, but use a grain of salt to take those daily numbers.

Rather, take the pictures "before" and "after" (or "progress"). You should compare them side by side down the line, to see how the body has changed over time. Photos can be a really motivational device because you may not note the small changes happening when you see yourself every day but when you compare pictures taken a month ago, the changes may be much more noticeable. Don't allow any current body dissatisfaction to stop you from taking pictures beforehand. You are going to be happy that you have them down the road.

In addition to the images, taking body measurements is useful. You can start building leaner muscle mass, particularly if you regularly work out or carry out strength training. You may not feel too much of a difference on the scale when your weight starts to change but your body composition may change dramatically. Measurements can help you track progress by tracking lost inches from various areas of your body. You will want to take the calculations below:

- Bust: weigh your bust all the way around, holding the measuring tape in line with your nipples.

- Chest: weigh your breasts or pectoral muscles immediately below and all the way down your back.

- Waist: find the narrowest portion of your waist, usually just below your ribcage, and weigh it all around.

- Hips: find and weigh the largest position of your hips all the way around.

- Thighs: weigh the whole round of the upper leg, when standing straight.

- Knees: weigh just above the knee all the way around, when standing straight.

- Upper arms: weigh the whole proportion of your upper arms above the elbows.

- Lower arms: weigh the entire part of your lower arms under your elbows.

You will need a non-stretchable measuring tape to properly measure. Hold the amount of tape across the body, parallel to the surface. Wrap the tape across your body as close to your skin as possible when you are measuring your measurements, but don't pinch so closely that the tape measure cuts into your skin or creates an indentation. Getting someone else taking your measurements for you is good so you can stand straight; if you don't have someone at your side, take your measurements in front of a mirror and make sure you keep the tape steady and weigh in the correct spots.

Make a list of your measurements in a notebook or notepad for your phone. Take the measurements every couple of weeks and log the numbers every time at the same location. You can use the metrics to track your progress as time goes on.

6.Expect Ups and Downs

Like anything in life, with intermittent fasting you'll experience ups and downs, particularly at the very start. Don't expect all to go right off the bat perfectly and don't get lost in glory. You'll slip up: sometimes you'll snack outside your feeding slot, and that's all right. If you go into it knowing you're trying to put your best foot forward but still realizing it can take a little while to get used to the change, you're going to be less likely to beat yourself up when things don't go absolutely according to schedule.

Chapter 3

What Do I Eat?

Nutrition isn't the idea of "one size fits all." Much as you would be ideally suited with a tailor-made wardrobe, a tailor-made diet plan will work well. That being said, there are some general concepts of nutrition you can use to figure out which foods are working for you and which ones are not. While the main goal of fasting is to go without eating for an extended period of time, eating healthy meals during your feeding periods is crucial as well. This will guarantee that you fulfill your nutritional needs and that you fuel the body with all the nutrients it needs to remain balanced and energized.

Choosing a Diet That's Right for You

Although the word diet is commonly associated with some type of food restriction, keep in mind that the actual definition of diet is "the type of food a person habitually consumes," and that's how you can understand the term here. There is no particular diet to adopt during intermittent fasting, but if you choose a diet full of nutrient-rich, unprocessed foods, you will of course reap the most benefits. Many diets are common supplements for intermittent fasting but do not get caught up in dogma. You need not follow a diet plan exactly as it was written. When you plan, for example, to follow a Paleo pattern but find that your body is doing well with brown rice, you should add it in. You don't have to skip a meal for good just because it doesn't come under the umbrella of a diet. Use intuitive eating to figure out the best possible approach.

Ketogenic Diet

One of the most popular dietary companions to intermittent fasting is the ketogenic diet. People who love intermittent fasting tend to lean towards this diet because the two approaches complement each other nicely: when combined, they will quickly kick you into a chronic ketosis (a physiological state where your body burns fat for energy rather than carbohydrates).

Most of your calories will come from fat when following a ketogenic diet and your carbohydrate consumption will be severely restricted. For comparison to other diets, a ketogenic diet allows you to keep track of just how much sugar, sugars, and protein you eat.

A typical ketogenic diet has a breakdown of the macronutrients:

- •60–75 percent of calories from fat

- •15–30 percent of calories from protein

- •5–10 percent of calories from carbohydrates

Low-Carb Diet

A low-carb diet is similar to a ketogenic diet in that you limit the daily intake of carbohydrates. A conventional low-carb diet, however, is not as high in fat, which requires a lower protein consumption than a ketogenic diet does. Most low-carb diets recommend an initial period of very low intake of carbohydrates— around two weeks — where you avoid nearly all foods containing carbohydrates, excluding low-carb vegetables. You'll lose a tremendous amount of water weight during this initial period. After these two weeks, you can move on to a more balanced plan where you can have healthier carbohydrate options, such as other grains, certain oranges, and whole-grain gluten-free. A standard low-carbohydrate diet's primary goal is to lower levels of blood sugar and leptin, and encourage weight loss.

Paleo Diet

The Paleo Diet is another common alternative to intermittent fasting, because it's built from your ancestors ' eating habits, including fasting. The basic concept of a Paleo Diet is to eat only items that were present during the Paleolithic era to hunters and gatherers. This description is, of course, open to interpretation because your Paleolithic ancestors wouldn't have access to things like almond butter cans, but you get the point.

You should eat, if you adopt a Paleo diet:

- Meat

- Fish

- Poultry

- Eggs

- Nuts and seeds

- Fruits

- Healthy fats (avocado oil, coconut oil, olive oil, ghee)

- Natural sweeteners (raw honey, maple syrup, coconut sugar)

- On the other hand, you'll need to avoid:

- Grains (wheat, oats, barley, rye, quinoa, couscous, amaranth, millet, corn)

- Dairy (milk, cheese, ice cream, butter)

- Legumes (soy, peanuts, chickpeas, beans)

- Alcohol

- Refined and artificial sweeteners (white sugar, high-fructose corn syrup, sucralose, aspartame

Pegan Diet

The Pegan Diet is a fairly new concept developed by Dr. Mark Hyman, the director of the Functional Medicine Center at Cleveland Clinic. The Pegan diet blends the basic principles of the Paleo diet with a vegan diet that seems counterintuitive, as at first glance the diets tend to be on the opposite ends of the spectrum; yet, their basic principles are very similar in reality.

Both the Paleo Diet and a vegan diet stress the option of whole, unprocessed foods which come from the land responsibly. The main differences are that the Paleo Diet relies on ethically sourced meats, beans, healthy fats, and some bananas, excluding both grains and legumes; a vegan diet excludes all animal products and incorporates wheat, legumes, herbs, and all plant-based foods. The Pegan diet's goal is to combine the two diets ' best things.

Approximately 75% of your daily intake must consist of plant-based foods using the Pegan diet. You will mostly want to eat vegetables; some fruits; some gluten-free grains, such as quinoa, brown rice and gluten-free oats; and some legumes, such as lentiles. The other 25% of your food intake should consist of high-quality animal proteins (grass-fed beef, pasture-grown chicken, and eggs) and healthy fats such as coconut, olives, and avocados (and their respective oils: coconut oil, olive oil, and avocado oil). Dr. Hyman recommends that meat be treated as a condiment rather than the main plant. Stick to 2–3 ounces of meat per meal, instead of a standard 4–6-ounce serving.

You must avoid gluten, meat, and some vegetable oils (canola, sunflower, corn, and soybean) while adopting a Pegan diet. Sugar— even natural forms such as honey and maple syrup— should only be consumed as an occasional treat. While natural sugars do provide some health benefits, overdoing them can have a negative impact on blood sugar levels — something you're ultimately trying to avoid when fasting intermittently.

Low-FODMAP Diet

FODMAPs, means fermentable oligosaccharides, disaccharides, monosaccharides, and polyols, are short-chain carbohydrates that may induce intestinal discomfort in those with digestive sensitivity. For someone who has chronic digestive disorder or unexplained irritable bowel syndrome, a low-FODMAP diet is typically recommended. When you eat a low-FODMAP diet, you'll stop other carbohydrate groups, including:

- •Oligosaccharides: oats, rice, legumes, garlic, onions, leeks, asparagus, jicama, fennel, beetroot, and Brussels sprouts

- •Disaccharides: white sugar, butter, yogurt, and soft cheeses such as cream cheese and cottage cheese

- •Monosaccharides: peaches, prunes, pears, nectarines, mangoes, watermelons, bananas, and honey

- •Polyols: blackberries, avocados, sweet potatoes, cauliflower, snow peas, and mushrooms

You'll eliminate all high-FODMAP foods for about a month after a low-FODMAP diet. You can reintroduce one high-FODMAP food at a time after this initial elimination period, to see how your body reacts. If you're not getting any digestive trouble, your stomach may be able to handle the food. If you do, you're likely sensitive to it, and you would do well to avoid it as much as you can.

Basic Nutrition Elements

For example, locking yourself into a certain food theory isn't appropriate. Basic nutrition principles (such as consuming only fresh, organic foods, eliminating processed foods and sugar, and eating plenty of fruits and vegetables) can be used to experiment with different types of foods to decide which foods perform for you and which foods you can avoid.

Grains

Grains are the hot topic quite a bit. It seems that specialists on agriculture–and the general population–are split in the middle when it comes to whether grains are good or bad for you. One side of the debate suggests eliminating grains, while the other side notes that whole grains are a must because of their value of fiber and vitamin B. So who's okay? Well, the answer is, it depends on that. The anti-grain side says there are three main grain problems: lectins, phytates, and gluten.

Lectins

Lectins are a type of protein found both in grains and legumes and binding to the membranes of cells. They are small and difficult to digest, because they are both heat and digestive resistant. Because of this, they tend to accumulate in your bloodstream and migrate all their way into your blood. Your immune system develops antibodies when proteins enter your blood as a whole, which means that it recognizes the protein as a foreign invader and builds up an attack against it. Over time this can lead to leaky intestines and increased sensitivity to lectins.

Phytates

Phytates are compounds found in grains and legumes, and in nuts and seeds in lower amounts. Phytates are not inherently bad for you, but they are often described as antinutrients because they bind to minerals such as iron, zinc, and calcium, preventing absorption of these. That can set you up for shortages in minerals. It's important to note here that phytates don't hinder the long-term ability to absorb nutrients; they only obstruct absorption at mealtime.

Gluten

Gluten is of course the most divisive when it comes to plants. Although celiac disease — an inability to digest gluten properly — is widely accepted, many people don't believe in the susceptibility of non-celiac gluten. Yet research shows that gluten can affect the lining of the intestines (and cause symptoms of celiac disease), even in people without the disease.

Scientists at the University of Maryland have discovered that your body produces a protein called zonulin when eating gluten. By developing gaps between the intestinal cells, which are normally extremely close, Zonulin negatively affects the gut lining. Food and microbes will move through them and reach the blood when these spaces are formed. Such ions activate an immune response once inside the blood that never gets shut off. This response can cause chronic disease and inflammation. Interestingly, it is the underlying factor in many autoimmune diseases. This is called "leaky gut" and recent evidence shows that gluten-consuming people have at least a mild form of it.

A Note on Wheat

Wheat has been part of farming for more than nine thousand years, and is one of the world's largest crops. It is considered an integral part of the food supply of many nations because it can be preserved for years in kernel form and can be refined to produce a wide variety of foods, including rice, breads, noodles, and cereals. The concern with wheat is not in the grain itself but what has been done to it by modern agriculture.

Today's wheat is not only lower in many of the nutrients that were historically in wheat, but the composition of the plant itself has improved due to modern milling. The aim of industrial technologies is to produce a crop that can thrive should tragedy occur, so it has become immune to disease, adverse weather, pests, and pesticides through major food companies. As a consequence, your body doesn't recognize wheat the way it used to. It's becoming toxic and addictive instead of offering nourishment.

Making Grains Healthier

If you want to add grains into your diet, there are a few items you can do to make sure the body better tolerates them. Next, select grains which are gluten-free. It is estimated that about 1 percent of the population suffers from celiac disease, while non-celiac gluten exposure is measured at up to 13 percent. Gluten allergy signs include:

- Bloating

- Constipation and/or diarrhea

- Abdominal pain

- Headaches

- Fatigue

- Skin problems (rashes, psoriasis, eczema, hives, dermatitis)

- Depression

- Unexplained weight loss

•Iron-deficiency anemia

•Anxiety

•Joint or muscle pain

•Autoimmune disorders

•Brain fog

Contains brown rice, wild rice, quinoa, buckwheat, millet, teff and amaranth. Oats are also technically gluten-free, but they're almost always contaminated by gluten due to the way they're made. If you wish to include oats in your diet, select brands specifically labeled gluten-free.

The next thing you can do is cook the grains before they are eaten. Soaking grains can help break down the phytats and neutralize the lectins, making the grains easier to digest and allowing you to absorb all the minerals inside. Place them in a bowl to soak the grains, and cover them with moist, filtered water. You must also add one tablespoon of an acidic medium, such as lemon juice or apple cider vinegar, for every cup of water that you add to the bowl. For starters, if you need to cover your grains with three cups of water, add three table spoons of lemon juice to the broth, and cover the bowl with a breathable medium, like a clean kitchen towel. First, let the kernels rest twelve hours. Rinse them off with cold water after the grains have soaked for an acceptable amount of time and continue with your preparation as planned.

Another option is to sprout your grains, or use already sprouted grains. Food manufacturers have caught up with the health benefits of sprouting their grains, and many businesses are now selling sprouting grains that can save you time and effort. If in the local grocery store you can't find sprouted grains, you can look online or sprout them yourself.

Sprinkling takes much longer than soaking grains, as you have to wait for the grain to actually crack open and form a sprout. Follow the soaking process to sprout your own grains, and then transfer the soaked and drained grains to a glass jar — a Mason jar works well. Place a cheesecloth over the container and allow the grains to stay in the moist jar for one to five days. When they're ready you'll learn, because the seeds will break open and a green sprout will be visible. The sprouted grains can be kept in the refrigerator for up to a week.

Dairy

Dairy is yet another controversial product in the world of nutrition. You've probably grown up hearing about how great your bones are in milk. The reality, milk isn't as healthy for your bones as you might imagine. In addition, the countries with the lowest intake of milk have the lowest fracture and osteoporosis levels, a disease in which the bones are fragile and are more likely to break and shatter. Furthermore, many people have difficulty digesting the proteins and sugars present in the milk. This is because when you mature, the production of lactase in your body—the enzyme you need to better digest milk—gradually declines.

That doesn't mean you can't eat any food either, but there are some choices that are safer than others. If you want to include milk in your diet, use milk that comes from grass-fed cows. Grass-fed milk, butter, and cheese are usually found at local stores. Unlike conventional dairy which has more omega-6s, grass-fed dairy has a higher omega-3 content. Omega-6s aren't inherently bad, but it can lead to chronic inflammation when you eat too many (which many Americans do). Cultivated grass-fed dairy products, such as yogurt and kefir, are also good choices, but note that they are full-fat and dry. Sweetened yogurts and kefirs are often loaded with sugar.

The goat's milk products are a great option if you want to skip cow's milk entirely. Current cow's milk contains high amounts of a protein called casein A1, which can be highly inflammatory (and exacerbate eczema and acne problems). Goat's milk, on the other hand, contains a protein called casein A2 which is not inflammatory. Studies show that people with A2 casein who drink milk reported decreased inflammation and no adverse digestive symptoms.

Meat and Poultry

Meat is another controversial food, vilified over the years because of its saturated-fat content. Before low-fat diets were truly popular, red meat was a big no - no; but since then, research has shown that saturated fat has less effect on heart disease than previously thought. The right forms of saturated fat will actually protect against heart disease.

The old school of thought was that saturated fat boosted cholesterol, which increased the risk of heart disease; but science now shows that while saturated fats will increase the amount of LDL in your blood, it produces the big, fluffy LDL particles that do not bind to the walls of the arteries. Saturated fat also increases levels of HDL and protects against heart disease.

Meat is one of vitamin B12's top sources, too. You can actually just get vitamin B12 from animal products. Meat also contains the remaining vitamins B, vitamin D, vitamin E, amino acids, antioxidants, and several minerals.

That said, it's important to choose high-quality, grass-fed meats just as with dairy. Conventional meat comes from GMO foods, cereals, and even sugar feeding calves. It fats the cows up faster to grow more but it also reduces their meat's nutritional content. Grass-fed meat also contains up to five times as many omega-3 fatty acids than regular beef and considerably fewer omega-6.

Grass-fed meat often contains a fat called the linoleic acid conjugated, or CLA. CLA acts as an antioxidant and has been shown to minimize the risk of heart disease, stop cancer tumor growth, prevent atherosclerosis, decrease triglycerides and decrease the risk of type 2 diabetes production. All animal foods contain some CLA, but grass-fed meat and dairy contain up to 500 per cent more than dairy and grain-fed meat from cows.

Not all poultry is the same, as beef. There's poultry originating from traditional farming and then there's poultry that's organically raised and allowed to roam freely, following a natural diet. You will often see poultry and egg labels that boast the birds were "fed a vegetarian diet," but chickens and turkeys are not vegetarians. They love scavenging for bugs, ticks and worms and that's what makes the chicken so nutritious. Poultry allowed to eat a naturally occurring diet is higher in omega-3s, vitamins and minerals.

When choosing poultry, choosing a combination of organic and raised pasture is the best option. If your local grocery store doesn't have this, or your budget doesn't allow it, talk to your local farmers. In your local farms, you may often find high-quality meat that is not branded raised pasture or organic (because these are government-moderated terms, and many small farms cannot afford to pay for the certification process required to carry such labels), but by nature these are both.

A Note on Eggs

There is much fear around cholesterol, so people often separate their eggs, throw away the yolk and eat only the white egg. While the egg white contains protein, most of the nutrients in an egg are present in its yolk, such as vitamin A, vitamin D, vitamin E, vitamin K, B vitamins, omega-3 fats, calcium and phosphorus. Do not be afraid of eating the entire egg, but choose the types of eggs that you consume wisely.

Many of the egg labels and nutrition claims are mere marketing tactics. The terms natural and farm new, for example, generally mean little. Other terms, such as cage-free, sound good but may be misleading. You might picture birds roaming outside in the sunlight when you hear the term cage-free, but cage-free just means the birds weren't in cages. We might still have been in a cramped factory without much room to move around. Organic and pasture raised are the best type of eggs that you can get. Once, talking to your favorite egg producers is a great way to find eggs of high quality that are typically fresher and less costly than the eggs that you will purchase in a grocery store.

Seafood

Seafood is loaded with protein and beneficial vitamins and minerals, but two specific omega-3 fatty acids: eicosapentaenoic acid (EPA) and docosahexaenoic acid (DHA) are the most notable health benefits linked to seafood. Regular use of EPA and DHA has been shown to increase the risk of heart disease, cancer, type 2 diabetes and autoimmune disease.

It is safer to eat fewer species of fish while picking the food. Larger fish higher on the food chain tend to accumulate more mercury in their flesh and other heavy metals and toxins.

The fish and shellfish that are highest in omega-3s include:

•Salmon

•Mackerel

•Trout

•Sardines

•Herring

•Oysters

•Mussels

When addition to selecting smaller fish rich when omega-3 fatty acids, it is also possible to choose fish that have been captured in the wild rather than raised in the farms. As with animals raised for conventional meat, farmed fish are fed a diet that is not theirs natural. This could include grain and corn. Farm-raised fish are rich in omega-6 fatty acids as a result of their unhealthy diet, and lower in omega-3 fatty acids. In addition, according to one study published in the Journal of the American Dietetic Association, it was not even possible to detect omega-3 fatty acids in some farmed fish sold in grocery stores. Farm-raised fish develop higher levels of toxins and chemicals in their food, in addition to altered levels of fatty acids.

Fruits and Vegetables

You think you are good at the fruits and vegetables. Of course, some fruit contains more natural sugar than others, but it is not a problem for most people when this sugar is combined with the fiber in the fruit. Problems arise from consuming too much fruit juice, which provides all the sugar without any of the nutrients, so be sure to eat it whole and preferably with the skin on (which includes fiber) while eating fruit.

Evidence has also shown that organic products contain not only less pesticides and herbicides than traditional products, but are also richer in certain vitamins and minerals. If your budget does not qualify for a lot of organic options, using the Dirty Dozen list of the Environmental Working Group, you should choose which fruits and vegetables to buy organic. The Dirty Dozen report outlines what usually have the most polluted fruits and vegetables. These are the things you can consider shopping organic products. The Dirty Dozen is:

- Strawberries

- Spinach

- Nectarines

- Apples

- Grapes

- Peaches

- Cherries

- Pears

- Tomatoes

- Celery

- Potatoes

- Sweet bell peppers

The Environmental Working Group also provides a list of the items, in addition to the Dirty Dozen report, which appears to have the lowest amount of chemicals and toxins. These are those fruits and vegetables you don't have to consider buying organic. This number is called the Clean Fifteen, and is the following:

- Avocados

•Sweet corn

•Pineapples

•Cabbage

•Onions

•Frozen sweet peas

•Papayas

•Asparagus

•Mangos

•Eggplant

•Honeydew melons

•Kiwis

•Cantaloupes

•Cauliflower

•Broccoli

Fats and Oils

Obesity is nothing to think about. In reality, it can provide useful vitamins and minerals, like healthy fats in your diet, and help to keep you full longer. The trick is to choose fats which are safe for you. Healthy, natural fats are vital components of a balanced diet.

Margarine contains hydrogenated oils which contain trans fats. Trans fats were developed to provide longer shelf-life for foods, but have a detrimental effect on cholesterol levels. Unlike saturated fats, which increase the large, fluffy LDL particles that don't stick to the walls of the artery, trans fats increase the thin, compact LDL particles that are trapped on the walls of the artery and can create blockages that increase your risk of heart condition.

Refined oils like soybean oil are rich in omega-6 fatty acids, which is a common ingredient in many prepackaged foods. Eating too many omega-6 fatty acids will, as you have already discovered, lead to chronic inflammation, which is related to a number of diseases and health problems.

The best fats to consume include:

- Olive oil

- Avocado oil

- Unsalted grass-fed butter

•Grass-fed ghee

•Coconut oil

•Walnut oil

•Hemp oil

•Sesame oil

Cooking with Fats

All fats have a certain level of smoke (a point at which they start smoking when exposed to some temperature). The cycle will break down some of the antioxidants and vitamins and even produce chemicals that are harmful to your health when the fats hit their smoke point. Care should be taken to cook only with oils that have a high point of smoke, particularly when using high heat. Avocado oil, honey, ghee, and coconut oil all have the highest points of smoke and are the easiest to eat. Olive oil can be used to cook but at low heat only. Walnut oil, hemp oil, and sesame oil are best used for dressing or healthy cooking.

Keeping the fats away from a heat source is also safest. When you store your fats right next to the pot, the leftover cooking heat will turn them rancid.

Sugar and Sweeteners

Most of the health issues often blamed on fat are actually due to sugar. Sugar has no health benefits, yet the average American consumes about 66 pounds of sugar per annum. The fact that sugar contributes to chronic inflammation, increases your risk of heart disease, destabilizes blood sugar levels, and feeds on cancer cells is even more worrying than having no nutritional value. Eating too much sugar can also make weight gain easier for you.

Manufacturers have tried to solve the sugar problem by marketing artificial sweeteners, but studies show that people who eat artificial sweeteners are at higher risk of diabetes, metabolic syndrome, and heart disease. Additionally, artificial sweeteners can throw off the bacterial equilibrium in your body, causing both digestive and neurological issues. We also related artificial sweeteners to cancer and chronic migraines. Besides that, if you give your body the sweet taste without any calories, it can induce even more extreme sugar cravings.

No matter what shape it is in, sugar should be as limited as possible. There are certain sweeteners for you, however, that are safer than others. The best options are to:

- Pure maple syrup

- Raw honey

- Coconut sugar

•Date sugar

•Monk fruit

•Molasses

•Stevia

•Erythritol

A Note on Stevia

While stevia is a plant and is sold as fresh, the moment it's available to you, many packaged types are highly processed. Besides that, some stevia products often contain added ingredients that are undesirable, such as "actual flavors." The word "natural flavors" is not closely regulated by the FDA, and even for chemical additives that mimic natural flavors, businesses are free to use this definition. If you choose stevia, do this sparingly, and make sure that you choose one that is pure and sustainable.

Fluids to take while fasting

While fasting only certain fluids can be consumed like; water, tea and coffee (hot or iced) and homemade broth.

1)WATER: The benefits of water cannot be overemphasized, so it important that you drink water frequently throughout the day when you fast. You can enjoy flat, mineral or carbonated water. You can add;

a)You can add lime

b)You can add lemon

c)You can add slices of other fruits (never eat the fruit or
  consume fruit juice)

d)You can add vinegar (raw, unfiltered apple cider vinegar
  is better)

e)You can add Himalayan salt

f)You can add Chia and ground flaxseed (mix one
  tablespoon in a cup of water)

g)You can add sweetened powders or drops

2)COFFEE: Consuming up to six cups of their caffeinated or
  decaffeinated coffee is allowed. Black coffee is preferable
  but you are only allowed to add 1 tablespoon of certain fats
  to each cup of coffee taken. You can also have a change by
  taking unsweetened iced coffee. Simply brew your coffee
  and then refrigerate it or add ice cubes.

  a)You can add coconut oil

  b)You can add medium chain triglyceride oil (MCT oil)

  c)You can add butter

d)You can add Ghee

e)You can add heavy whipping cream (35% fat)

f)You can add half and half milk

g)You can add whole milk

h)You can add ground cinnamon, for flavor

i)Try and avoid low fat or skimmed milk; whole milk is preferable

j)You can add powdered dairy products

k)You can add natural or artificial sweeteners of your choice

3)HERBAL TEA: There is no limit as to the number of herbal tea you can consume during your fasting period. There quite a number of herbal teas that can help suppress your appetite and lower your blood sugar levels.

a)Green tea: This serves as a good appetite suppressant

b)Cinnamon Chai tea: This helps to lower the blood sugar levels and it is also good for suppressing cravings of sweet food.

c)Peppermint tea: This acts as a good appetite suppressant. It helps with alleviating GI discomfort such as gas and bloating.

d)Bitter melon tea: It helps to lower blood sugar levels

e)Oolong tea: This also helps to lower blood sugar levels

Black tea is preferable but you are only allowed to add 1 tablespoon of certain fats to each cup of coffee taken. You can also have a change by taking unsweetened iced coffee. Simply brew your coffee and then refrigerate it or add ice cubes.

a)You can add coconut oil

b)You can add medium chain triglyceride oil (MCT oil)

c)You can add butter

d)You can add Ghee

e)You can add heavy whipping cream (35% fat)

f)You can add half and half milk

g)You can add whole milk

h)You can add ground cinnamon, for flavor

i)Try and avoid low fat or skimmed milk; whole milk is preferable

j)You can add powdered dairy products

k)You can add natural or artificial sweeteners of your choice

4)HOME MADE BROTH: It is normal if you experience some lightheadedness during the first few days of fasting. This is caused by dehydration and low levels of electrolytes and it can reduce by taking a good homemade broth. Both vegetable and broth made with meat, fish or bones will work. Bone broth is very beneficial because it contain an important ingredient called gelatin which is very good for people suffering from arthritis or other joint problems. There is no limit as to the amount of broth you can consume during the fasting day.

a)You can mix any vegetable that goes above the ground

b)You can take leafy vegetables

c)Carrots

d)Onions or shallots

e)Bitter melon

f)Animal meat

g)Animal bones

h)Fish meat

i)Fish bones

j)Himalayan salt

k)Any dried or fresh herbs and spices

l)One tablespoon of ground flaxseed per cup

m)Vegetable puree of any kind

n)Potatoes, yam, beets or turnips

o)Always avoid any store bought broths even though they
    are organic

Chapter 4

Exercise And Training During Intermittent Fasting

A lot of women are going to see success by themselves with intermittent fasting. During certain windows they do a good job of eating, and when they eat they ensure that their food is full of nutrition. But if you want to improve your results and burn extra fat then adding some workouts to your routine is important. This chapter will look at the steps you will take to prepare and exercise properly while you are on the sporadic fast.

Nevertheless, a recent study undertaken by a Swedish Institute of Sport and Health Sciences showed that reducing the overall amount of carbohydrates in your diet helps the body to more efficiently burn calories and improve the muscle growth potential. Ten elite level cyclists went through an hour of interval training in this study, going at about 64 percent of their aerobic maximum capacity. They either had low or normal glycogen muscle levels that were attained prior to diet or exercise intervention.

Ten muscle biopsies were taken prior to training, about three hours after the workout was completed. The results showed that exercise has been able to increase mitochondrial biogenesis while in a glycogen-depleted state. This is the mechanism whereby new mitochondria will develop within the cells. The authors of the study conclude that exercise on a diet low in glycogen may be helpful in enhancing oxidative muscle ability. Part of what makes working out when you're already in a fasted state is that the body has some processes that help preserve and protect the muscles from losing themselves. So, if you're low in fuel for a workout, which you'll of course be when you're on an intermittent fast, your body will start breaking down some of the other tissues, but not the active muscle you're using.

Exercising while preserving your muscles

Many experts agree about 80 percent of your health benefits from a healthy lifestyle come from your diet. The rest comes from exercise. This means that if you actually want to lose weight you need to focus on eating the right foods. It is important to realize, however, that both exercise and eating well are essential.

Researchers studied data from 11 participants on the "The Biggest Loser" show. The participants ' total body fat, total energy expenditure, and resting metabolic rate were measured three times. These were measured after six weeks at the start of the programme, then at 30 weeks. Using a human metabolic model, the researchers were able to quantify the influence of changes in diet and exercise resulting in weight loss to see how both led to this target.

Researchers found that most weight loss was attributable to diet alone. Just about 65 percent of this weight loss was from body fat, however. The rest of the body weight reduction stemmed from lean muscle mass. Exercise alone only resulted in fat loss and a slight increase in lean muscle mass.

Exercising and fasting together

If you're trying to get an effective exercise program that adds some high intensity training as well as intermittent fasting, there are a couple of components that need to come together. Whether you like you don't have enough energy to keep on with the exercises when you do this then it's time to make a change. Reducing the number of hours you are fasting for usually will make a difference. Intermittent fasting is meant to make you feel great, and if not, then the time has come to change your plan.

There are two main points to keep in mind while you work out while you're on the sporadic hard. The first one concerns the timing of your meals. Intermittent fasting isn't all about extreme restrictions on calories. You're not meant to deprive yourself to great results. Instead, it's just a matter of timing the meals well so you don't binge for most of the day. You may eat in a small window, maybe in the evening or later part of the day. So if you restrict your evening meal to just 4 and 7, you'll be fasting for 21 hours.

Ranging from 12 to 18 hours of fasting is suitable for most men. Many people prefer to run for 16 hours, as this is the fastest time to fit into their busy schedules. You will figure out what works best for your needs by making sure you get all the benefits.

If you have trouble abstaining entirely from food during the day, then you want to restrict your dinner to a small portion of sweet, low-glycemic food. These include healthy options every four to six hours, such as poached eggs, whey protein, vegetables and fruit. Any days you choose to sleep, it's best to avoid having at least three hours of food before going to bed. Doing this will help minimize your system's oxidative damage and can really make it easier to achieve intermittent fasting.

Additionally, on the days you work out you should break your fasts with a recovery meal. On the days you need to exercise while fasting, you need to eat a recovery meal about 30 minutes after you've finished working out. Adding whey protein to your diet easily assimilates will aid improve muscle recovery.

It's a good idea to fast again after you've had that meal, until you eat your main meal that night. After each workout session it is important to eat a proper recovery meal. This will ensure your body gets the energy it needs, and that there is no muscle or brain damage. Do not skip this meal, and make sure you get it after the workout within 30 minutes.

If you think it's hard to do fasting for 12 to 18 hours, you can get the same results from exercise and fasting by skipping breakfast and running right in the morning when you're having an empty stomach. This is because eating a large meal before a workout, particularly one that is carb-heavy, inhibits the sympathetic nervous system and reduces the effects of your exercise on fat burning.

While most people have been taught to take a lot of carbs in before a workout in order to get endurance and see results, this works against the goals you have. Eating too many carbs stimulates the parasympathetic nervous system which promotes energy storage and inside the body stores calories and carbs. This is probably the last thing you expect if you are running and on the hard irregular, so it is easier to see better results soon.

Tips for getting the most out of your workouts

It's not supposed to be hard to work out on an irregular easy. Exercise and plenty of physical movement are intended to help you feel good, muscle building and weight loss. Some of the ways you can make sure you're doing really well while training on an irregular fast include:

- Start slow— if you've never completed a weightlifting program before, you'll need to start slowly. Even if you're just returning to an ongoing exercise routine, acknowledging the improvements you've made is crucial and doing it slowly so you know how they will affect your results.

- Add more weight when you feel comfortable— if you start to feel comfortable, it's important to consistently add more weights. With time, the weights with which you continue your exercise will begin to feel pretty light, and if you don't make any changes, you'll see the performance slowing. This does not mean that you want to force your body past its limits, but it does mean that if you hope to see continued success, you will want to increase the difficulty of your exercise routine on a regular basis.

- More reps and more weight is better for lean muscles-If you're looking for lean muscle construction, try doing less repetitions at higher weights. This can drain the body more efficiently and will deliver better outcomes.

•Don't forget to warm up and cool down–Just because you
need to change your eating habits doesn't give you an
excuse to leave out the warm-up and cool down parts of
your workout schedule. Take at least five minutes at
exercise start and end to stretch the muscles not only will
improve performance, it will also reduce the likelihood of
injury.

•Keep on shape— we're sometimes too focused on how
much weight we can carry while we work out at the gym.
It's actually more important to have proper form, however.
Instead of adding more weight and doing it poorly, it is
better to do an exercise with the right form with less
weight.

Social And Life Benefits Of Intermittent Fasting

1.Time: When you worry less about having to constantly interrupt your routine to have a meal you will be surprise as to how much time you have to do other things. Intermittent fasting gives you more time to focus on other things without distractions.

2.It helps you save money: When you don't have to spend money on panic eating you tend to spend less. You might be consuming the same amount of calories but when you concentrate on a meal a day you will save more.

3.It makes traveling easier: When you travel to different countries you won't worry about the diet choices you have to make. This gives you more room and protects you from fat gain and encourages nutrient partitioning.

4.It increases your stamina: Intermittent fasting is solely based on the unlimited fatty acids that are store in the body therefore your stamina is increased tremendously. Once your body has gotten used to fasting you won't have the fear of running out of energy.

5.Admiration: Not everyone might appreciate the steps you are taking but I can guarantee that some of your friends and family will admire your incredible self-control. This boosts your ego and makes you feel very good.

6. It increases your will power: Intermittent fasting doesn't require much will power as it is easy to do. Sticking to it makes you have a feeling of self-control and accomplishment. Research has shown that achieving control and success in one area strengthens you will power in other aspects of your life.

7. It helps to avoid ego depletion: While you are on intermittent fasting you tend to make less food decisions during the course of the day which in turn saves you from fatigue and ego depletion. Research has shown that decision making drains your energy reserves and this reduces your decision making ability.

8. It helps you to understand the difference between appetite and hunger: With intermittent fasting you have better clarity when it comes to a whimsy appetite in contrast to actual hunger. This helps you to understand need vs. want which I quite revolutionary and empowering.

9. It helps you to lose the hunger fear: Intermittent fasting makes you have control over your ravenous appetite. The longer you fast the less hungry you become. This will help you to stop planning snacks or when you are going to eat.

10.It helps you to enjoy food without any guilt or restriction:
Intermittent fasting is ta good solution to easy weight loss
without the feeling of guilt or restriction. During
intermittent fasting you can eat without feeling guilty and
still burn all the stubborn areas of fat.

Increase Energy And Improve Your Life Quality

1)Control stress

The feelings triggered by stress eat enormous amounts of energy. Talking to a friend or family, attending a support group or seeing a psychotherapist can all help to make depression more difficult. Relaxation techniques such as mediation, self-hypnosis, yoga and tai chi are also effective tools for stress reduction.

2)Lighten your load

Overwork is one of the main reasons for tiredness. Academic, family and social responsibilities may include overwork. Consider streamlining your "must-do" task list. Set priorities for the most important tasks. Pare down the less important ones. If need be, consider asking for additional help at work.

3)Exercise

Exercise is almost guaranteed to make you sleep better. It also gives the cells more burning energy, so oxygen circulates. And exercising causes the release of epinephrine and norepinephrine in your body, stress hormones that can make you feel energized in modest amounts. Even a brisk walk is a good beginning.

4)Avoid smoking

Smoking poses a threat to your safety. But you may not realize that your vitality is potentially siphoned off by smoking inducing insomnia. Tobacco nicotine is a stimulant, thereby accelerating heart rate, increasing blood pressure and enhancing wakefulness-related brain-wave function, making it difficult to fall asleep. And once you fall asleep, with cravings, its addictive strength will kick you in and wake you up.

5)Restrict your sleep

When you think you may be deprived of sleep, seek to get less sleep. This suggestion can sound strange because deciding how much sleep you really need will reduce the amount of time you waste not lying in bed. This cycle makes it easier to fall asleep and long-term encourages more restful sleep. Here's how to do it:

•Stop a morning napping.

•The first night, go to bed later than usual, and sleep for just four hours.

•If you like you've been sleeping well during that four-hour period, add another 15–30 minutes of sleep the following night.

•As soon as you're soundly asleep the whole time you're in bed, keep steadily applying more to the nights that follow.

The 21 Day Guide For Fast And Easy Weight Loss

Day 1

BREAKFAST

- Breakfast Casserole

You can prepare this delicious casserole in advance a day or two so you'll have a quick breakfast ready to go that doesn't require any extra preparation.

Ingredients

- 1 pound 85 percent lean ground beef

- 1 small yellow onion, peeled and diced

- 1 teaspoon freshly ground black pepper

- 1 teaspoon garlic powder

- 1 teaspoon red pepper flakes

- 12 large eggs

- •1 cup unsweetened full-fat coconut milk

- •1 tablespoon coconut oil

- •1 small butternut squash, peeled, seeded, and sliced

Preparation

- •Start cooking ground beef in a large skillet over medium heat. Add onion and spices and simmer for 10 minutes until the onions are tender.

- •Whip the eggs and the milk together in a large bowl.

- •Grease 4–6 quarter slow cooker with coconut oil inside. Put in a combination of peas, beef and onions, and egg and milk. Stir and ensure that the beef and onion mixture is completely covered with a mixture of egg and milk. Cook for 10 hours, on low heat.

- •Mix, slice, and serve warm.

LUNCH

- •Roasted Beet Slaw

New beets are versatile, flavorful, and nutritious, but use the root bulbs not only.

Ingredients

- 1 teaspoon sea salt

- 3 large beets, scrubbed

- 2 tablespoons olive oil

- ¼ cup balsamic vinegar

- 3 cups thinly sliced bitter beet greens

- ¼ cup raisins

- 1 teaspoon toasted pine nuts

- ¼ teaspoon salt

- ¼ teaspoon freshly cracked black peppercorns

Preparation

- Preheat a 350 ° F boiler.

- Sprinkle the salt of the sea on an unfrozen pan. Toss the beets in the oil and put them on the salt bed; roast until the beets are fork-tender for about 1 hour.

- Heat the vinegar in a large sauté pan over medium heat for 1 minute while the beets roast. Attach greens and raisins; heat for about 3 minutes until greens are wilted and raisins have plumped up a little.

•Remove the beets from the oven, cut and thinly slice them when cool enough. In a medium bowl, mix sliced beets, vegetables, raisins and pine nuts; season with salt and pepper, and serve.

DINNER

•Lamb Patties

The lamb may be served fresh to medium-rare but the egg should be cooked thoroughly. Fruit chutneys or chia seed jams match meat patties well.

Ingredients

•1 medium shallot, peeled and minced

•2 cloves garlic, peeled and minced

•½ pound ground lamb

•1 egg white

•¼ cup dried currants

•¼ cup whole pistachio nuts

•½ teaspoon ground cinnamon

•¼ teaspoon freshly cracked black peppercorns

•1/8 teaspoon salt

Preparation

•Preheat oven to 350 degrees F.

•Mix the shallots and garlic with the lamb, cabbage, currants, cinnamon and nuts. Season with salt and pepper.

•Blend into 6 small ovals. Place in a baking dish of 8 ' or 8 ' and bake for 15 minutes. Serving hot.

Day 2

BREAKFAST

•Autumn Breakfast Chia Bowl

This fall-reminiscent Autumn Breakfast Chia Bowl features cranberry and cinnamon flavors but it can be enjoyed any time of year.

Ingredients

- •3 cups cold water

- •1/4 teaspoon salt

- •1 cup gluten-free steel-cut oats

- •1/2 cup unsweetened almond milk

- •3 tablespoons chia seeds

- •1 tablespoon halved macadamia nuts

- •1 tablespoon raw sliced almonds

- •1/2 teaspoon ground cinnamon

- •1 tablespoon no-sugar-added dried cranberries

Preparation

- •Bring water and salt to a boil over high heat in a medium saucepan, then add the oats. Reduce heat to medium-low, stir and add milk.

- •Apply the seeds of chia, the nuts of macadamia, the almonds, cinnamon and cranberries and mix.

- •Cover and cook for 20 minutes on medium-low heat, stirring occasionally until the chia seeds become soft and gel-like. Serve straightaway.

LUNCH

- •Spicy Shrimp with Lemon Yogurt on Wilted Greens

Prepare this delicious lemon yogurt a day beforehand and you're never going to wonder how to dress up your shrimp again.

Ingredients

- •1 cup organic, grass-fed, full-fat plain yogurt

- •¼ cup fresh lemon zest

- •6 cups bitter greens

- •12 large shrimp (approximately ½ pound), peeled and deveined, tails on

- •1 teaspoon olive oil

- •2 cloves garlic, peeled

- •¼ teaspoon freshly cracked black peppercorns

- •¼ cup thinly sliced black olives

- •1 medium lemon, thinly sliced

Preparation

- •Prepare yogurt sauce by combining yogurt and zest together, then cover over night and refrigerate.

- •Wilt greens in a steamer, about 4 minutes, then instantly chill in the refrigerator, about 10 minutes.

- •Butterfly shrimp by cutting almost but not completely through the middle of the tail, instead pressing halves down to form a butterfly pattern.

- •Brush the shrimp in a large bowl of butter, garlic and pepper. Switch to large skillet and cook for 5 minutes over medium heat until the shrimp has turned white and pink and is firm to the touch.

•Put greens on serving plates in mounds, then add the shrimp. Lemon yogurt and dollop on top of shrimp. Sprinkle with olives on each serving, and garnish with lemon slices.

DINNER

•Lentil-Stuffed Peppers

Those Lentil-Stuffed Peppers are as leftovers even better. Make them in advance and store them for a quick meal in your fridge, ready to eat when you're ready to break your fast.

Ingredients

•1 tablespoon olive oil

•2 medium yellow onions, peeled and finely diced

•2 stalks celery, finely diced

•2 large carrots, peeled and finely diced

•4 cups vegetable stock, divided

•3 cups dried red lentils

•6 medium red bell peppers, tops cut off and set aside, seeds and ribs removed

•6 sprigs fresh oregano, tops reserved and remaining leaves chopped

•3 ounces feta cheese

•¼ teaspoon freshly cracked black peppercorns

Preparation

•Heat oil over medium heat in a large saucepan for 1 minute. Stir in onions, celery and carrots; sauté for 5 minutes, then add 1 cup of vegetable stock and lentils. Simmer for 20 minutes, before fully cooked lentils.

•Put the bell peppers in a big, shallow 3 cup pot of vegetable stock. Cover for 10 minutes and boil, then remove from heat.

•Put the lentils, oregano, feta and black pepper together in a bowl; put the spoon into bell peppers.

•Ajar peppers with stem tops to eat. Garnish with oregano tops which are reserved.

Day 3

BREAKFAST

•Turkey, Egg White, and Hash Brown Bake

With this satisfying dish you can beat any cravings for a hearty but still healthy breakfast. Quick and easy to whip, this bake is perfect for the day's first meal – or any meal.

Ingredients

•Olive oil cooking spray

•1 tablespoon olive oil

•1 pound 85 percent lean ground turkey

•1 pound Russet potatoes, peeled and shredded

•12 large eggs

•11/2 teaspoons salt

•11/2 teaspoons freshly ground black pepper

•1/2 teaspoon ground cayenne pepper

Preparation

•Preheat oven to 375 degrees F.

- Grease a 9'x 13' glass cooking spray casserole bowl.

- Heat oil in a pan for 1 minute over medium heat. Add the ground turkey and cook for about 6 minutes, until no longer pink.

- Transfer cooked turkey to a large bowl and use the remaining ingredients to combine. Blend well.

- Pour the mixture into baked pot. Bake for 40 minutes until top is set, and a toothpick inserted comes out clean.

- Allow 5 minutes to settle, then break in 16 pieces and serve.

LUNCH

- Traditional Greek Salad

Salads are an excellent way to boost the consumption of vegetables after a fasting regimen. Don't be afraid to pile your daily intake of micronutrients on any vegetables you want.

Ingredients

- ½ head iceberg lettuce, trimmed, cored, and torn into bite-sized pieces

- ½ head romaine, trimmed, cored, and torn into bite-sized pieces

- 1 medium red onion, peeled and sliced

- 1 medium cucumber, sliced

- 2 small beefsteak tomatoes, quartered

- ¼ bunch fresh oregano, chopped and stems discarded

- ¼ cup extra-virgin olive oil

- 3/4 cup red wine vinegar

- ¼ teaspoon freshly cracked black peppercorns

- 6 ounces feta cheese, crumbled

- 2 ounces jarred pepperoncini

- 6 anchovy fillets

- ½ cup cured Greek olives

Preparation

- Construct salad by layering the lettuces and vegetables on a serving platter or in a large bowl.

- Blend oregano with sugar, vinegar and black pepper in a small bowl to create dressing.

•Drizzle salad dressing. Finish with crumbled feta, anchovies, pepperoncini and olives.

DINNER

•Mustard green beans

Ingredients

- •1 pound green beans, trimmed

- •1 tablespoon extra-virgin olive oil

- •1 tablespoon mustard (any kind)

- •Himalayan salt and ground black pepper

Prep time: 10 minutes

Cook time: 10 minutes

Yield: 4 servings

Preparation

•Fill a medium sized casserole with ample water to cover the green beans and bring to a boil over medium to high heat. Attach the beans and boil for around 3 to 4 minutes, until crisp and tender. Instead, the beans can be steamed: fill a casserole with water about three-quarters full and add a basket of steamer on top. At medium-high heat bring the water to a boil. Add the beans to the steamer basket and steam for about 5 minutes, until crisp and soft. Take off fire.

•Heat the olive oil over medium heat in a non-stick skillet for 5 minutes, before adding the mustard.

•Add the cooked beans to the mixture of oil and mustard and cook for about 2 minutes, until well combined and warm.

•Remove the beans from the skillet, season with salt and pepper as needed and serve;

Day 4

BREAKFAST

•Cran-Orange Oatmeal

If you feel a bit bland about your standard oatmeal recipe, try this revamped version! Add extra vitamins and minerals to tart cranberries and fresh orange — and a zesty flavor that turns things up a notch.

Ingredients

•1 cup freshly squeezed orange juice

•1/2 cup water

•1 cup fresh cranberries

•2 cups gluten-free rolled oats

•1 tablespoon maple syrup

•1 tablespoon freshly grated orange zest

Preparation

•In a medium saucepan, mix orange juice, sugar, and cranberries over medium heat. Take for about 5 minutes to a boil.

•Apply oats and boil, stirring continuously and for about 8 minutes before thickened. Stir in maple syrup and remove from heat.

•Divide the oatmeal into two bowls, garnish and serve immediately with orange zest.

LUNCH

•Carrot Thyme Soup

Try adding a sweet potato to the soup if your carrots aren't "sweet enough" Peel the potato, dice it into small squares, then add the other ingredients to the stockpot.

Ingredients

•2 pounds large carrots, peeled and diced

•1 large Vidalia onion, peeled and diced

•4 red potatoes, peeled and diced

•3 cloves garlic, peeled and minced

•1 tablespoon olive oil

•6 cups vegetable stock

•4 sprigs fresh thyme, stems removed

•¼ teaspoon salt

•¼ teaspoon freshly cracked black peppercorns

Preparation

•Put carrots, cabbage, potatoes and garlic with oil in large
stockpot. Sweat steadily, around 10 minutes over
medium heat.

•Remove stock and bring to a boil; cook uncovered for
about 1 hour.

•Remove the mixture from the heat and allow to cool
slowly, around 5 minutes, then purée until smooth in a
blender.

•Return the purée to the pot and add thyme, salt and
pepper; simmer 30 minutes uncovered over low heat.
Spoon in and drink in pots.

DINNER

•Roasted cauliflower rice

Ingredients

•1 head cauliflower

•½ tablespoon Himalayan salt

Prep time: 10 minutes

Cook time: 15 minutes

Yield: 2 servings

Preparation

- •Preheat the oven to 200°F. Line a baking sheet with parchment paper.

- •Cut the cauliflower into florets and remove the stems.

- •Grate the cauliflower by hand or pulse it in a food processor until it looks like rice.

- •Spread the cauliflower rice on the prepared baking sheet and sprinkle with the salt.

- •Place the baking sheet in the oven and bake for 12 to 15 minutes, flipping every 5 minutes.

- •Remove before the cauliflower rice starts to brown.

- •Add any desired herbs or spices.

Day 5

BREAKFAST

•South of the Border Scrambler

Short on schedule? This version of scrambled huevos rancheros can be made in minutes. If you are looking for a pop, spice it up with some sliced jalapenos.

Ingredients

•4 large eggs

•1/2 teaspoon salt

•1/4 teaspoon freshly ground black pepper

•1 teaspoon olive oil

•1/4 cup no-sugar-added salsa

•1/2 large avocado, diced

•1/4 cup chopped fresh cilantro

Preparation

•In medium bowl, whisk the beans, salt, and pepper together.

•Steam the olive oil over medium heat for 30 seconds in a small skillet. Add the eggs and scramble for about 4 minutes, until fried.

•Move to two cups, with 1/8 cup salsa, 1/4 diced avocado and 1/8 cup cilantro in each.

•Serve straightaway.

LUNCH

•Escarole with Rich Poultry Broth

Escarole is a leafy green which belongs to the chicory family. You can replace endive, chicory, or kale as well.

Ingredients

•1 tablespoon olive oil

•3 pounds skinless, bone-in chicken

•2 large yellow onions, peeled and sliced

•4 cloves garlic, peeled and minced

•1 cup dry red wine

•3 quarts no-sugar-added chicken stock

- •1 bunch fresh flat-leaf parsley, chopped and stems discarded

- •½ bunch fresh thyme, chopped and stems discarded

- •3 dried bay leaves

- •10 black peppercorns

- •¼ teaspoon salt

- •2 bunches escarole, trimmed and cored

Preparation

- •Heat oil in a medium-sized stockpot over medium heat. Attach chicken, onions, and garlic; sauté for about 10 minutes, until chicken is golden brown.

- •Pour in wine and allow to reduce by half, cooking over low heat, uncovered for about 7 minutes. Add stock, and simmer 2 1/2 hours uncovered.

- •Apply spices and peppercorns to the saucepan and steam for another 30 minutes. Season with salt, then drain and put the broth aside. During the next stage reserve chicken on a plate to cool.

- •Steam cut, cored escarole in steamer for about 5 minutes, until it was barely wilted. Place the escarole into the bottom of serving bowls and ladle in broth to serve.

•Cut and remove bones from chicken once the chicken has cooled, then add chicken meat to soup bowls.

DINNER

•Avocado fries

Ingredients

•2 large avocados, cut into ¼ -inch-thick slices

•Juice of ½ lime

•1 cup pork rinds

•1 tablespoon Himalayan salt

•Dried herbs and/or spices

•1 egg

•2 tablespoon melted coconut oil or butter

Prep time: 15 minutes

Cook time: 15 minutes

Yield: 4 servings

Preparation

•Preheat the oven to 400°F.

•Place the pork rinds in a sealable plastic bag and crush
    with your hands until they resemble bread crumbs. Mix
    in the salt and any other dried spices or herbs.

•Pour the lime juice into a small bowl. In a separate small
    bowl, whisk the egg.

•Dip each avocado slice first in the lime juice, then in the
    egg. Let sit in the egg for about 10 seconds, then flip to
    coat the other side of the slice.

•Place the egg-coated avocado slices in the bag with the
    crushed pork rinds and shake until the slices are
    covered in the pork rind mixture.

•Pour the melted coconut oil into a baking dish and place
    the avocado slices in the dish.

•Cook for 15 minutes, or until golden brown.

Day 6

BREAKFAST

- Tomato Spinach Frittata Muffins

Easy to bake, and fun! Eat frittata with those muffins in a new way.

Ingredients

- 2 cups finely chopped fresh spinach
- 11/2 cups halved cherry tomatoes
- 1 scallion, trimmed and finely chopped, green part only
- 10 large eggs
- 2 tablespoons unsweetened full-fat coconut milk
- 1 teaspoon dried ground oregano
- 1/8 teaspoon salt
- 1/4 teaspoon freshly ground black pepper

Preparation

- Preheat oven to 375 degrees F. Grease cooking spray into a 12-cup muffin pan.

•Divide the spinach, tomatoes and scallion evenly and place them in cups of muffin.

•Whisk the eggs, milk, oregano, salt and pepper together in a medium saucepan. Equally dump the egg mixture into each cup of muffins.

•Bake the eggs for 20 minutes until they are fully set. Serve.

LUNCH

•Dandelion and White Bean Soup

Dandelions are not only weeds-they are nutrient-rich greens filled with antioxidants, vitamin K, vitamin C and vitamin A!

Ingredients

•1 teaspoon olive oil

•2 medium yellow onions, peeled and chopped

•3 medium carrots, peeled and diced

•3 stalks celery, diced

•4 cloves garlic, peeled and minced

•2 quarts vegetable stock

- 1 dried bay leaf

- ¼ bunch fresh flat-leaf parsley, chopped and stems discarded

- 4 sprigs fresh thyme, stems discarded and leaves chopped

- ¼ teaspoon freshly cracked black peppercorns

- 2 cups fresh dandelion greens

- 1 cup cooked cannellini beans

- ¼ cup freshly grated Romano or Parmesan cheese

Preparation

- Heat oil over medium heat in a large stockpot for 1 minute. Remove the onions, carrots, celery, and garlic; sauté for about 4 minutes until light brown.

- Add stock and simmer uncovered for 1 1/2 hours at low heat.

- Apply herbs and spices to the pot; cook 30 minutes more uncovered.

- Steam dandelion greens for about 7 minutes in a steamer, until al dente. Attach greens and beans to soup; cook for 15 minutes, uncovered.

- In cooking bowls ladle broth and top with cheese.

DINNER

•Tomato, cucumber, and avocado salad

Ingredients

  •2 cups diced cucumbers (about 1 medium cucumber)

  •1 cup halved cherry tomatoes

  •1½ cups cubed avocado (about 1 large avocado)

  •1 cup green olives, pitted and halved

  •½ cup feta cheese

  •1 tablespoon balsamic vinegar

  •4 tablespoons extra-virgin olive oil

  •½ teaspoon freshly ground black pepper

  •1 teaspoon Himalayan salt

Prep time: 15 minutes

Yield: 2 servings

Preparation

•Toss the cucumbers, onions, avocado, and olives together in a medium sized dish.

•Sprinkle it over the feta cheese.

•Garnish with balsamic vinegar and olive oil on top and toss.

•Apply salt and pepper to taste.

Day 7

BREAKFAST

•Flourless Banana Cinnamon Pancakes

These pancakes are the simplest and healthiest you'll ever produce. These are gluten-free and contain ingredients which you possibly already have on hand.

Ingredients

  •1 large egg

  •1/2 ripe medium banana, mashed well

  •1 teaspoon chia seeds

  •1 teaspoon ground cinnamon

  •1 tablespoon coconut oil

Ingredients

  •Blend potato, banana, chia seeds and cinnamon in a large glass, measuring cup or blender at low speed, until smooth.

  •Heat the oil over medium heat in a small skillet. Pour two little circles of flour onto the skillet and cook for about 4 minutes, until bubbly on top and golden on bottom. Flip over and cook for 2 minutes. Repeat on batter left over.

LUNCH

•Wild Rice Salad with Mushrooms and Almonds

This is a vegetarian dish but try sautéed shrimp or diced baked chicken breast if you want.

Ingredients

•¼ cup yellow raisins

•1 cup filtered water

•1 cup uncooked wild rice

•3 cups water, lightly salted

•1 cup whole raw almonds

•1 tablespoon extra-virgin olive oil

•8 ounces shiitake mushrooms, sliced

•¼ teaspoon salt

•¼ teaspoon freshly ground black pepper

•2 scallions, trimmed and chopped

•1 teaspoon ground cumin

•Juice of 1 medium lemon (about 2 tablespoons)

Preparation

- •Soak the raisins in 1 cup of hot water for 30 minutes until overnight.

- •Boil wild rice in a medium saucepan over high heat in partially salted water until most grains burst open, around 35 minutes. Wash and wash.

- •Lightly toast almonds over medium heat in a dry small skillet until most of them have thin, dark brown spots and achieve an oily shine, around 5 minutes. Place the almonds on a plate to cool until room temperature, around 10 minutes.

- •Heat the oil over high heat in a medium skillet for 1 minute, then cook the mushrooms for about 5 minutes until tender. Season with salt and pepper.

- •Mix rice, almonds, mushrooms (with cooking oil), raisins, and scallions in a mixing bowl. Deposit back.

- •Toast cumin in a warm, small skillet for about 3 minutes, until fragrant. Take off fire.

•Toss rice bowl mixed with lemon juice and toasted cumin. Serve at room temperature, or cold.

DINNER

•Strawberry and kale salad

Ingredients

   •4 cups kale

   •12 strawberries, diced

   •1 cup walnuts

   •1 tablespoon balsamic vinegar

   •4 tablespoons extra-virgin olive oil

   •Himalayan salt and ground black pepper

Prep time: 10 minutes

Yield: 2 servings

Preparation

•Toss the kale, strawberries, and walnuts together in a large bowl.

•Spoon the salad over the vinegar and the olive oil.

•Season with salt and pepper, if needed.

DAY 8

BREAKFAST

•Coconut Cacao Hazelnut Smoothie Bowl

This delicious nutty and chocolaty bowl is loaded with healthy fats and micronutrients. Enjoy it as your firstmeal of the day to get your daily nutrient needs off to a jump start.

Ingredients

•1 tablespoon shredded unsweetened coconut

•1 cup unsweetened almond milk

•1 frozen ripe medium banana

•2 teaspoons raw unsweetened cacao powder

•1½ teaspoons pure maple syrup

•1/8 teaspoon sea salt

•6 ice cubes (approximately 1/2 cup)

•5 hazelnuts, shelled and chopped

•1 tablespoon shelled pumpkin seeds

Preparation

•Toast coconut over medium heat in a small skillet, stirring often until the flakes are golden brown, about 3 minutes. Deposit aside.

•To mix with cream, add milk, banana, cacao, maple syrup and salt and blend until smooth. When you wish to make the mixture thicker add more ice.

•Garnish with hazelnuts, pumpkin seeds and toasted coconut in a serving bowl and top. Serve.

LUNCH

•Warm Spinach Salad with Potatoes, Red Onions, and Kalamata Olives

Use this basic, tasty dish as a master recipe: a starting point from which to produce myriad of your own variations!

Ingredients

•10 cups fresh curly leaf spinach, washed, stems removed

•1 pound small red potatoes, scrubbed and cut into 1/2' slices

•¼ cup extra-virgin olive oil

•1 medium red onion, peeled, halved, and thinly sliced

•20 Kalamata olives, pitted

•1 tablespoon balsamic vinegar

•¼ teaspoon salt

•¼ teaspoon freshly ground black pepper

•

Preparation

•In a large mixing bowl, add spinach leaves.

•In a medium pot, boil potatoes 10 minutes on high heat. Drain.

•Heat olive oil in a large skillet over high heat 1 minute. Add potatoes and onion and cook until potatoes are slightly browned, about 5 minutes. Remove from heat; add olives, vinegar, salt, and pepper.

•Pour potato mixture over spinach and invert skillet over bowl to hold in heat. Allow to steam 1 minute. Divide onto four plates, arranging potatoes, onions, and olives on top. Serve warm.

DINNER

•Pear and arugula salad with pine nuts

Ingredients

- 4 cups arugula

- 1 pear, thinly sliced

- ½ cup pine nuts

- ½ lemon

- 4 tablespoons extra-virgin olive oil

- Himalayan salt and ground black pepper

Prep time: 10 minutes

Yield: 2 servings

Preparation

- Toss the arugula, pear slices, and pine nuts together in a large bowl.

- Squeeze the lemon juice halfway over the salad.

- Pour the olive oil onto the salad.

- Season as desired with salt and pepper.

Day 9

BREAKFAST

•Overnight Almond Butter Pumpkin Spice Oats

You'll love digging into these nutritious and hearty pumpkin oats! This recipe is great for a busy day at tidying you up.

Ingredients

•½ cup gluten-free rolled oats

•¼ cup unsweetened almond milk

•¼ cup pumpkin purée

•½ teaspoon pumpkin pie spice

•½ teaspoon alcohol-free vanilla extract

•½ teaspoon ground cinnamon

•1 tablespoon pure maple syrup

•2 tablespoons unsalted, no-sugar-added almond butter

•2 tablespoons chopped walnuts

Preparation

•Mix the oats and milk in a medium bowl, and whisk. Add the purée of pumpkin, the spice of pumpkin pie, vanilla, cinnamon and maple syrup. Delete.

•Pour half a mixture of oats into two small canned jars each. In each glass, add 1 spoonful of almond butter over oats. Divide the excess almond butter over the remaining oats. Fill with lids on pot. Chill overnight.

•Top with walnuts in the morning, and enjoy! The combination can be chilled for up to 3 days.

LUNCH

•Lentil Salad

Lentils are rich in carbohydrates but their high fiber content slows down digestion, which can help to balance sugar and energy in the body. This delicious Lentil Salad is an outstanding way to quickly interrupt your overnight stay.

Ingredients

•1 pound dried lentils, washed, undesirables discarded

•2 quarts lightly salted water

•2 medium yellow onions, peeled and finely chopped

- 3 scallions, trimmed and chopped

- 1 medium green bell pepper, stemmed, seeded, and finely chopped

- 1 tablespoon cumin powder

- 1/8 teaspoon cayenne pepper

- Juice of 1 medium lemon (about ¼ cup)

- 2 tablespoons extra-virgin olive oil

- ¼ teaspoon salt

- ¼ teaspoon freshly ground black pepper

Preparation

- Boil lentils over high heat in a medium saucepan of water until soft but not split, about 12 minutes. Place over a plate for 5 minutes to cool.

- Mix the lentils in a large bowl with the onions, scallions and green pepper.

- Toast cumin in a hot, dry skillet for about 3 minutes, until fragrant. Take off fire.

•Apply cumin and remaining ingredients to the lentil mixture and serve in a cup.

DINNER

•Arugula and prosciutto salad

Ingredients

•2–3 cups arugula, washed

•6–9 thin slices of prosciutto

•½ cup chopped tomato

•½ cup sliced olives

For the dressing

•1 tablespoon extra-virgin olive oil

•1 teaspoon balsamic vinegar

Prep time: 10 min

Yield: 1 serving

Preparation

•Toss together the arugula, prosciutto, tomato and olives in a medium-sized bowl.

•Make the sauce: Blend olive oil and vinegar together.

•Place the salad over the dressing, or eat the side dressing.

Day 10

BREAKFAST

- Mini Quiche

These promise a delicious protein-packed breakfast — or any meal of the day — and can be made to last in bulk for the week.

Ingredients

- 6 large eggs

- 6 slices nitrate- and nitrite-free bacon

- 1 tablespoon pure olive oil

- ½ cup chopped fresh broccoli florets

- ½ cup sliced white mushrooms

- ½ cup peeled and diced yellow onions

- ½ cup seeded and diced red bell peppers

Preparation

- Preheat oven to 325 degrees F. Fill tinned muffin with 8 cups of foil.

- Whisk the eggs together, then set aside.

- Fry the bacon until it is crisp, about 5 minutes, then let the paper towel cool for 5 minutes, before chopping in ½ bits.

- Add the oil over medium - high heat to the medium sauté tray. Stir in remaining ingredients for 5 minutes.

- Pour the eggs into foil cups, filling 2/3 of the way into each cup.

- Only split bacon and vegetables into each cup.

- Cook until golden brown, for 25 minutes. Serve.

LUNCH

- California Garden Salad with Avocado and Sprouts

The fruity taste of large green Florida avocados adds a brighter, more summery feel to this salad than the original California Hass avocado.

Ingredients

Dressing

- 1 tablespoon freshly squeezed lemon juice

- 3 tablespoons extra-virgin olive oil

- •1 tablespoon finely chopped shallot

- •½ teaspoon salt

- •¼ teaspoon freshly ground black pepper

Salad

- •2 heads Boston or Bibb lettuce, trimmed and cored

- •2 large ripe beefsteak tomatoes, cored and cut into 8 wedges each

- •1 ripe medium avocado, peeled, pitted, and cut into 8 wedges

- •1 cup alfalfa sprouts

Preparation

- •Mix lemon juice, olive oil, shallot, salt and pepper in a small bowl, and blend properly.

- •Make salad: place leaves of lettuce, the stem ends in, on four bowls, make a petal pattern for the fruit. Within leaves are going to be too low so save them for another use.

- •Toss tomatoes in 1 spoonful of dressing; place 4 tomato wedges on each salad. Toss the avocado with another 1 liter of dressing; put 2 wedges of avocado on each salad. Divide sprouts between slabs. Drizzle the remaining salads with the sauce, or serve on the table.

DINNER

•Steak fajitas

Ingredients

   •2 tablespoons butter, divided

   •1 red bell pepper, thinly sliced

   •1 green bell pepper, thinly sliced

   •1 yellow bell pepper, thinly sliced

   •½ onion, chopped

   •1 tablespoon Himalayan salt

   •½ teaspoon freshly ground black pepper

   •1 pound skirt steak

   •Large leaves of Boston lettuce (or other lettuce), for serving

   •For topping (this is optional)

•Sour cream

•Guacamole

•Pico de gallo

•Lime wedges

•Grated cheddar cheese

Prep time: 10 minutes

Cook time: 20 minutes

Yield: 2 to 4 servings

Preparation

•Heat a big skillet, apply medium-heat. Melt 1 spoonful of butter in the pan.

•Remove the onion and bell peppers, then season with salt and pepper. Turn on food. Stirring occasionally, for 15 to 20 minutes, until the peppers are tender.

•If the vegetables have to cook for about 10 minutes, fire a second large skillet over medium heat. Melt the remaining butter spoon in the pan.

•When the vegetables are left to cook for about 10 minutes, season the steak with salt and pepper and place it in the butter skillet. Cook, until seared, for 3 to 5 minutes at each side.

•Take both skillets off oil.

•The steak will rest 5 to 10 minutes before slicing. Cut into desired thickening pieces.

•Slice the steak and vegetables into 2 to 4 equal parts and cover each part in a broad leaf of lettuce. Apply the fajita toppings you like and enjoy.

Day 11

BREAKFAST

•Spicy Kale Scramble

This great breakfast after workout provides healthy proteins and greens-with a kick!

Ingredients

- •1 tablespoon olive oil

- •1 cup chopped fresh kale

- •3 large eggs, whisked

- •2 teaspoons ground turmeric

- •½ teaspoon salt

- •¼ teaspoon freshly ground black pepper

- •1/8 teaspoon ground cayenne pepper

Preparation

- •Heat the olive oil over medium heat in a medium skillet for 1 minute. Add the kale and cook for about 3 minutes, before wilted.

•Apply the whisked eggs and remaining ingredients to skillet. Scramble the eggs for about 4 minutes, until cooked clean.

•Serve immediately.

LUNCH

•Pumpkin Soup with Caraway Seeds

Butternut squash, or even acorn squash, in this soup very well substitutes for pumpkin. Each of them imparts their own style, transforming all three recipes into one. Chipotle or Spanish paprika (both sold in gourmet stores) incorporate a faint smokiness and add an extra layer to flavor.

Ingredients

•2 tablespoons unsalted grass-fed butter

•1 medium yellow onion, peeled and chopped

•1 large carrot, peeled and thinly sliced

•2 cups peeled and cubed pumpkin

•¼ teaspoon whole caraway seeds

•1½ cups vegetable stock

•3 cups unsweetened full-fat coconut milk, divided

•¼ teaspoon salt

•¼ teaspoon freshly ground black pepper

•½ teaspoon dried chipotle chili pepper

Preparation

•Melt butter over medium heat for 1 minute in a big, heavy-bottomed soup pot. Add the onion, carrot, pumpkin, and caraway seeds; sauté, stirring occasionally, for 10 minutes until pumpkin becomes tender and starts to brown (some may stick to pan).

•Covered 20 minutes of stock and simmer. Remove from heat and stir in the milk in 2 cups.

•Puree soup in batches until creamy in a blender, changing consistency with the remaining milk. Mix with pepper and salt. Sprinkle on top of chipotle chili pepper or Spanish paprika for garnish.

DINNER

•Homemade chicken fingers

Ingredients

- •1 pound of boneless chicken breasts, trimmed to 1 inch wide by 3 inches long

- •2 eggs

- •1 cup of crushed pork rinds/cracklings

- •1 tablespoon of Himalayan salt

- •1 teaspoon of freshly ground black pepper

- •1 teaspoon of smoked paprika

- •1 teaspoon of garlic salt (this is optional)

- •2 tablespoons of coconut oil

- •Hot sauce, for serving (this is optional)

Prep time: 10 minutes

Cook time: 20 to 30 minutes

Yield: 2 servings

Preparation

- •Preheat the oven to 300°F. Line a baking sheet with aluminum foil.

- •Wash the chicken fingers and pat dry.

•In a small bowl, combine the crushed rinds of pork, salt, pepper, smoked paprika, and garlic (if used). Pour right into a sealable plastic bag when mixed.

•Bat the eggs in a medium-sized tub. Dip each chicken finger to coat in the eggs.

•Apply the egg-coated chicken fingers and the spice mixture to the container.

•Seal and shake the chicken is coated in a bag.

•Put the chicken fingers onto the baking sheet and put them in the oven.

•Bake 10-15 minutes.

•Turn the chicken over and cook until golden brown for another 10 to 15 minutes.

•Remove the chicken from the oven and allow to cool for 5 minutes.

•If desired, serve with hot sauce.

Day 12

BREAKFAST

- Vegetarian Hash

An old favorite's version explodes of flavor. As a side dish or as an entry, it can be served.

Ingredients

- 1½ pounds Russet potatoes, peeled and large-diced

- 1 medium poblano (or other mild chili pepper), halved and seeded

- 2 medium red bell peppers, stemmed, halved, and seeded

- 1 medium red onion, peeled and thickly sliced

- 1/2 teaspoon olive oil

- 1 tablespoon chili powder

- ¼ teaspoon freshly cracked black peppercorns

- ¼ bunch fresh cilantro, chopped

- ¼ teaspoon salt

Preparation

- Preheat oven to about 400 ° F.

- Toss the butter with the tomatoes, beans, and onions and dump onto a plate. Place vegetables on an unfrozen baking sheet and season with chili powder and black pepper; roast to a fork tenderloin. (Varying times; fork search at5-minute intervals)

- Large-dice peppers and onions. Combine tomatoes, beans, cilantro and onions. Cover and drink with salt.

LUNCH

- Smooth Cauliflower Soup with Coriander

It's easy on metabolism because this soup is purée. Eating this creamy dish as your first meal after your fasting period should help kick your digestion gradually and lighten your body into the afternoon.

Ingredients

- 2 tablespoons unsalted grass-fed butter

- 1 medium yellow onion, peeled and diced

- 2 tablespoons white wine

- •1 large head (about 2 pounds) cauliflower, cored and cut into bite-sized pieces

- •2 cups vegetable stock

- •1 teaspoon salt

- •¼ teaspoon ground white pepper

- •1 teaspoon ground coriander

- •¾ cup unsweetened full-fat coconut milk, divided

- •¼ teaspoon chopped fresh chives

Preparation

- •Melt butter over medium to high heat in a large saucepan or soup pot for 1 minute. Remove onion; cook until translucent but not dark, for about 5 minutes.

- •Pour in wine and cauliflower; simmer for 1 minute to steam alcohol. Remove the stock, salt, pepper, and coriander; carry over high heat to a rolling boil, then change to low heat.

- •Let the mixture boil for about 15 minutes, until the cauliflower is very tender. Switch to a mixer. Add half milk and purée until it is very creamy, scraping with a rubber spatula down the sides of the blender. Be very careful during this step because if not gradually started, hot liquids will splash out of the blender (you might want to purée in two lots, for safety).

•If necessary, switch soup back to casserole and thin with extra milk. Just before eating garnish with chopped herbs.

DINNER

•Gameday wings

Ingredients

•2 pounds of chicken wings

•1 tablespoon Himalayan salt

•1 teaspoon freshly ground black pepper

•1 tablespoon baking powder

•1 teaspoon smoked paprika

•1 teaspoon garlic salt (this is optional)

•2 tablespoons coconut oil

•2 tablespoons hot sauce (this is optional)

Prep time: 5 minutes

Cook time: About 20 minutes

Yield: 2 pounds of wings

Ingredients

- •Wash the chicken wings and pat dry.

- •Mix the salt, pepper, baking powder, paprika and garlic (if used) in a small bowl.

- •Place the wings in plastic sealable bag and apply the spice mixture. Seal the bag to coat the wings and shake.

- •Preheat the squash over medium heat. Melt the coconut oil in the hot saucepan.

- •Put the wings and coat them in the skillet. Cook for about 10-12 minutes.

- •Flip the wings and cook, until golden brown, for another 10 to 12 minutes.

- •Remove the heat from the wings and allow to cool for 5 minutes.

- •Spray hot sauce on the wings, if desired.

Day 13

BREAKFAST

•Chicken Sausage Patties

These tasty sausages go well with a side of Vegetarian Hash and poached eggs.

Ingredients

•3 pounds ground chicken

•1 medium yellow onion, peeled and finely minced

•½ cup finely chopped fresh flat-leaf parsley

•1 tablespoon chopped fresh sage (or 2 teaspoons dry ground sage)

•6 cloves garlic, peeled and minced

•1 tablespoon peeled and minced fresh ginger (or 2 teaspoons dry ground ginger)

•2 teaspoons red pepper flakes

•1 teaspoon ground cloves

•1 teaspoon ground white pepper

•4 tablespoons olive oil

Preparation

•Combine all ingredients in a large mixing bowl; stir well
by hand.

•Approximately 2 ' round mixture into 24 patties.

•In a small sauté pan, heat the oil until hot, about 30
seconds. Stir patties on each side over medium heat for
about 5 minutes, until cooked through.

LUNCH

•Vichyssoise (Potato and Leek Soup)

This soup is comfortable and easy to prepare, and will leave
you full and satisfied. If you incorporate a low-carbohydrate
diet into your fasting plan, this recipe can be adjusted using
turnips in place of potatoes. Replace the potatoes with equal
quantities of turnips and prepare likewise.

Ingredients

•1 tablespoon olive oil

•1 medium yellow onion, peeled and chopped

- •1 pound (about 4 medium) potatoes, any variety, peeled and cut into 1' chunks

- •2 bunches leeks, washed twice, chopped, and divided

- •1 teaspoon dried sage

- •1 bay leaf

- •¼ cup white wine

- •2 quarts vegetable stock

- •¼ teaspoon salt

- •¼ teaspoon ground white pepper

Preparation

- •Heat olive oil in a large saucepan over medium heat for 1 minute. Add cabbage, carrots, and all but 1 bunch leeks; boil for 10 minutes until translucent ointments. Add experience, leaf of port, and wine. Cook an extra minute.

- •Remove pot stock. Bring to a full boil on high heat, then reduce to low heat and cook for 45 minutes until the potatoes are very tender and begin to fall apart.

•Carefully purée the broth in small batches in a blender. Season with white pepper and salt.

•Steam, boil or sauté 1 bunch of leeks in the middle of each pot, about 4 minutes, and serve soup garnished with a spoonful of leeks.

DINNER

•Chicken stuffed bell peppers

Ingredients

•1 tablespoon butter

•1 clove garlic, minced

•1 small onion, diced

•1 teaspoon Himalayan salt

•½ teaspoon freshly ground black pepper

•1 teaspoon smoked paprika

•1 teaspoon chili powder

•1 cup grape tomatoes, halved

•1 pound ground chicken

- •3 eggs, beaten

- •4 large bell peppers, halved

Prep time: 10 minutes

Cook time: 1 hour 30 minutes

Yield: 4 servings

Preparation

- •Preheat the oven to 350°F. Line a baking sheet with parchment paper.

- •Melt butter over medium heat in skillet. Remove the chili powder, ginger, onion, oil, pepper, paprika. Cook for five to seven minutes.

- •Pour in the tomatoes and sauté 5 to 7 minutes more.

- •Remove chicken to the ground and cook until golden brown, stirring occasionally for about 15 minutes.

- •Move the mixture of cooked meat to a medium sized bowl and gently pour in the eggs.

- •Lay half cut side up onto the prepared baking sheet with each bell pepper. Pour the bell peppers into the meat and egg mixture.

•Place the stuffed peppers in the oven and bake until the peppers soften slightly, for 60 minutes.

Day 14

BREAKFAST

- Artichoke and Cheese Squares

These rich vegetable cakes are easy to prepare and can be prepared 3 days in advance.

Ingredients

- 1 (12-ounce) jar marinated artichoke hearts, drained and chopped, liquid reserved

- 1 small yellow onion, peeled and finely chopped

- 2 cloves garlic, peeled and finely minced

- 4 large eggs, beaten

- 2 tablespoons coconut flour

- ½ teaspoon salt

- ¼ teaspoon freshly ground black pepper

- ¼ teaspoon dried ground oregano

- ¼ teaspoon Tabasco

•8 ounces shredded Monterey jack cheese

•2 tablespoons chopped fresh flat-leaf parsley

Preparation

•Preheat oven to 325 ° F.

•In a small skillet, flame artichoke liquid over medium heat
for 1 minute. Stir in skillet onion and garlic for 5
minutes until translucent onions.

•Blend potatoes, rice, salt, pepper, oregano and Tabasco in
a mixing bowl. Combine cheese, parsley, artichokes,
garlic and onion.

•Pour the mixture into a baking dish of 7' or 11.' Bake until
the egg is ready for 30 minutes. Nice for ten minutes.
Cut into squares and drink at room temperature, or
warm up at 325 ° F for 10 minutes.

LUNCH

•Chickpeas in Potato Onion Curry

If you come home starving and nothing is ready for dinner,
thirty-minute main dishes like this are a lifesaver. Put on a pot
of brown rice to eat with it before you continue this dish and
you will dine before you know it.

Ingredients

- •2 large yellow onions, peeled and cut into 1' pieces

- •3 tablespoons olive oil, divided

- •1½ cups peeled and cubed (1' pieces) Russet potatoes

- •1 (13.5-ounce) can unsweetened full-fat coconut milk

- •1 (15-ounce) can chickpeas (garbanzo beans), drained and rinsed

- •6 cloves garlic, peeled

- •1 teaspoon salt

- •1½ teaspoons ground coriander

- •½ teaspoon ground turmeric

- •1 teaspoon chili powder

- •1 teaspoon ground cumin

- •Juice of ½ medium lemon

Preparation

•Fry the onions in 1 tablespoon of oil in a large skillet over high heat until lightly browned, about 5 minutes. Add potatoes and milk; cover and cook for about 20 minutes, until the potatoes are tender. Attach the chickpeas and may to low heat.

•Combine the garlic, salt, coriander, turmeric, chili powder and cumin in a food processor; process until the mixture becomes a paste, scraping the processor sides as necessary.

•Heat the remaining oil in a medium skillet and fry for 1 minute until slightly browned and fragrant.

•Add the potato mixture to the cooked paste. Simmer on for 3 minutes. Spray with, and drink with lemon juice.

DINNER

•Chicken drumsticks wrapped in bacon

Ingredients

•4 chicken drumsticks

•4 slices bacon

•1½ teaspoons Himalayan salt

•1 teaspoon freshly ground black pepper

Prep time: 5 minutes

Cook time: 45 minutes

Yield: 2 servings

Preparation

- •Preheat the oven to 400°F. Line a baking sheet with aluminum foil.

- •Wrap one piece of bacon around each drumstick, working your way from the bottom of the drumstick to the top. Place on the prepared baking sheet and season with the salt and pepper.

- •Bake for 45 minutes, or until the bacon looks nice and crispy.

Day 15

BREAKFAST

•Roasted Vegetable Frittata

This Roasted Vegetable Frittata can be prepared ahead of time and served at room temperature just above. It is the perfect way to use any remaining vegetables, so do not hesitate to be creative with anything in your refrigerator.

Ingredients

- •1 medium zucchini, quartered lengthwise and cut into chunks

- •1 medium yellow squash, quartered lengthwise

- •1 cup small white mushrooms, roughly chopped

- •1 small Italian eggplant (or 1/4 a regular eggplant), cut into large chunks

- •2 tablespoons olive oil

- •9 large eggs, beaten

- •3/4 cup unsweetened almond milk

- •1/2 teaspoon salt

- 2 tablespoons unsalted grass-fed butter

- 1 medium Russet potato, peeled, baked and diced

- 1 medium yellow onion, peeled and chopped

- 1 tablespoon chopped fresh flat-leaf parsley

- ½ cup diced tomato (about 1 large)

- 1 cup shredded cheese (Monterey jack, Cheddar, or Havarti)

- ¼ teaspoon freshly ground black pepper

Preparation

- Preheat 400 ° F oven. Toss courgettes, yellow squash, mushrooms, and olive oil eggplant together.

- Pour the mixture over an unfrozen baking sheet or in a roasting pan. Roast in the oven for about 20 minutes, until tender. Cut the mixture from the vegetables and increase oven temperature to 450 ° F.

- Whisk together eggs, milk and salt in a medium saucepan. Melt butter over medium heat in an oven-safe, 12 "nonstick skillet, about 20 seconds.

- •Add potatoes, onions, and parsley to skillet; cook for about 10 minutes until the onions are softened and the potatoes are slightly browned.

- •Add to the pan roasted vegetables and egg mixture. Cook, stirring with a wooden spoon, about 4 minutes until the mixture begins thickening but remains largely liquid.

- •Garnish with tomatoes and cheese. Season with pepper. Place the pan on the middle oven rack and bake until the frittata puffs slightly and start browning on top, around 15 minutes.

- •Remove the skillet from the oven and place the frittata on the serving platter. Enable it to rest for 5 minutes before cutting and serving to 8 wedges.

LUNCH

- •Red Pepper Soup

The few drops of vanilla enhance this delicious soup's savory flavors. Serve it warm in winter — without the toppings — or cool in summer months, as described.

Ingredients

- •1 tablespoon olive oil

- •3 medium red bell peppers, stemmed, seeded, and diced

- •1 large red potato, peeled and diced

- •1 cup peeled and diced carrots

- •1 large parsnip, peeled and diced

- •6 cups water

- •¼ teaspoon sea salt

- •1/8 teaspoon freshly ground black pepper

- •1/8 teaspoon alcohol-free vanilla extract

- •¾ cup canned unsweetened full-fat coconut milk, refrigerated

- •¼ cup chopped fresh chives, divided

Preparation

- •Heat oil in a large stockpot over medium to low heat for 1 minute.

- •Place the vegetables in a bowl and sauté for 10 minutes. Add some water. Bring to a boil at high heat, then switch to low heat and simmer 3 hours uncovered until vegetables are very tender. Season with pepper and salt.

Stir in some coffee. Remove from heat and allow to cool, around 15 minutes.

•When cold, in batch purée soup in a food processor or blender, until it is completely smooth.

•Divide the broth into six single serving cups. Swirl into each bowl 2 table spoons of milk and sprinkle with the chives.

DINNER

•Chicken "breaded" in pork rinds

Ingredients

•1¼ cup pork rinds

•1 tablespoon Himalayan salt

•2 teaspoons freshly ground pepper

•2 teaspoons smoked paprika

•4 chicken thighs, skin on

•2 large eggs

Prep time: 15 minutes

Cook time: 45 minutes

Yield: 2 servings

Preparations

•The oven should be heated to 375 ° F. Line aluminum foil on a baking sheet.

•Put the rinds of pork in a sealable plastic bag and break them with your hands until they imitate the crumbs of bread. In the pork rinds, add the salt, pepper and smoked paprika and shake until the spices and pork rinds are thoroughly mixed.

•Whisk the eggs in a small saucepan.

•In the egg mixture, place one of the chicken thighs and leave in for 10 seconds.

•Put the egg-coated chicken thigh and crushed pork rinds and seasonings into the container. Shake on the prepared baking sheet until the thigh is powdered, then pick and put on.

•Repeat with chicken thighs remaining.

•In the oven, put the baking sheet and cook for 45 minutes, or until golden brown.

Day 16

BREAKFAST

•Tomato and Leek Frittata

Leeks give to this frittata a mild flavor but you can also use onions in their place. For an added flair, eat this frittata, garnished with fresh goat cheese, tomato slices, and scallions.

Ingredients

•3 teaspoons olive oil, divided

•½ cup chopped leek greens

•½ teaspoon sea salt, divided

•½ teaspoon freshly ground black pepper, divided

•½ cup whole grape tomatoes

•¼ cup capers, drained and rinsed

•3 egg whites

•1 teaspoon dried herbes de Provence

•1 teaspoon dried thyme

•2 egg yolks

•2 ounces goat cheese, crumbled

Preparation

•Preheat a 350 ° F boiler.

•Heat 2 teaspoons of oil over medium heat in a 10' oven-
    safe skillet for 1 minute. To the pan, add leeks, 1/4
    teaspoon salt and 1/4 teaspoon pepper. Cook on for 5
    minutes.

•Pour the tomatoes and capers into the wine. Cover and
    cook for 3 minutes. Mixture moved to a small bowl.

•Rapidly beat egg whites with Provence spices, thyme, and
    remaining salt and pepper in a medium bowl. In egg
    yolks, stir until the mixture is moist.

•Spray the remaining skillet with grease. Add seasoned
    eggs, mixture of cooked tomatoes and cheese of goats.
    Cook for 4 minutes over medium heat.

•Switch the skillet to the oven; bake until the eggs are
    ready for 20 minutes. Cut a small slit in the middle of
    frittata for inspection. Chop and drink.

LUNCH

Chicken Piccata

This lunchtime treat (or at any time!) is a great blend of protein, lemon zest and artichokes.

Ingredients

- 1 cup no-salt-added chicken broth

- ½ cup freshly squeezed lemon juice

- 4 skinless, boneless chicken breasts

- 3 tablespoons olive oil

- 1 cup chopped yellow onion

- 1 clove garlic, minced

- 2 cups chopped fresh artichoke hearts

- 3 tablespoons capers

- 1 teaspoon pepper

Preparation

- In a shallow dish, add chicken broth, lemon juice and chicken to taste. Cover and marinate at refrigerator overnight.

•Heat the olive oil 30 seconds over medium heat in a
saucepan, then add the onion and garlic and cook for
about 2 minutes until softened.

•Save the chicken from the marinade, marinade stocks.
Add the chicken to the pan and brown on each side, for
a total of 8 minutes.

•Add core artichoke, capers, pepper and marinade
reserved. Reduce heat to low and simmer for about 10
minutes, before chicken is thoroughly cooked.

DINNER

•Grain-free cauliflower pizza

Ingredients

•1½ cups cauliflower florets (about 1 pound)

•2 large eggs, lightly beaten

•1 teaspoon Himalayan salt

•1 teaspoon dried oregano

•1 teaspoon garlic powder

•Pizza toppings of your choice

Prep time: 10 minutes

Cook time: 30 to 35 minutes

Yield: 1 8-inch pizza (about 3 servings)

Preparation

- Preheat the oven to 400°F. Line a baking sheet with parchment paper.

- Pulse the flowering cauliflower in a food processor until finely chopped. Transfer to big bowl.

- Remove and blend well the whites, salt, oregano and garlic powder.

- Move the mixture of cauliflower to the middle of the prepared baking sheet and use your hands to make it into a pizza crust.

- Cook for about 20 minutes, or until white.

- Apply the toppings you want and bake for another 10 to 15 minutes

Day 17

BREAKFAST

•Raspberry Banana Mint Chia Pudding

Raspberry and mint make this pudding perfect for breakfast — or any time of the day!

Ingredients

•½ cup canned unsweetened full-fat coconut milk

•½ cup unsweetened almond milk

•¼ cup chia seeds

•1 teaspoon alcohol-free mint extract

•1 tablespoon pure maple syrup

•1/2 ripe medium banana, sliced

•10 fresh raspberries

•2 tablespoons shredded unsweetened coconut

•2 whole fresh mint leaves

Preparation

•In a pot, add the milk, chia seeds, mint extract and maple
syrup and blend well. Cover and refrigerate, blend every
2 hours during the day, then cool overnight.

•Apply slices of banana to jar, supplemented by
raspberries, coconut and mint leaves. Right away
indulge or refrigerate for up to 2 days.

LUNCH

•Shredded Chicken Wraps

Lettuce wraps are a great way without the sugars to get the feel
of a tortilla wrap. To change the menu you can easily replace
your favorite meat or fish with the chicken.

Ingredients

•2 boneless, skinless chicken breasts, baked and shredded

•2 stalks celery, chopped

•¼ cup chopped fresh basil

•2 tablespoons olive oil

•2 tablespoons freshly squeezed lemon juice

•1 teaspoon peeled minced garlic

•1/8 teaspoon freshly ground black pepper

•1 head radicchio

•Mix chicken in a large bowl with celery, basil, olive oil, lemon juice, garlic, and pepper.

•Separate radicchio lettuce leaves and place on 8 plates.

•Spoon chicken mixture onto lettuce leaves and roll up.

Preparation

•Blend the chicken with the celery, basil, olive oil, lemon juice, garlic and pepper in a large bowl.

•Separate leaves of radicchio lettuce, on 8 pots.

•Chicken spoon paste on leaves of lettuce and roll up.

DINNER

•Simple homemade bacon

Ingredients

•2 pounds of pork belly

•2/3 cup Himalayan salt

•2 tablespoons freshly ground black pepper

•Any dried herbs and spices (this is optional)

Prep time: 15 minutes, plus 5 to 7 days to cure and 12 hours to chill

Cook time: 1½ to 2 hours

Yield: 2 pounds of bacon

Preparation

•Use a very sharp knife to remove skin from the pork belly. Try to keep the skin intact, as you remove it in one piece.

•Rinse the pork belly with a paper towel, and pat dry.

•Mix the salt, the pepper and any dried herbs and spices in a small bowl. Fry the pork belly on both sides of the mixture.

•Put the pork belly inside an airtight sealed container and refrigerate for 5 to 7 days. The stronger the flavour, the longer you cure it. Flip daily over the pork belly. (See to wash your hands thoroughly before you touch your pork belly.)

•Remove the pork belly from the fridge after 5 to 7 days and clean it off with salt, pepper and any other herbs and spices. Dry Pat.

•Oven preheat to 90 ° C (200 ° F).

•Put the rack in a roasting pan. Place fat side up the pork belly on the rack.

•Cook until the interior temperature of the meat exceeds 150 ° F. It normally takes an hour and a half to two hours to finish.

•Remove from the oven the pork belly and allow to cool for 30 minutes.

•Pack the meat in a parchment paper and place in the refrigerator for 12 hours or overnight.

•Slice the beef over a sharp knife to the desired thickness. You can now fry your organic bacon, or lock it in the refrigerator for up to 5 days, or up to 2 months in the freezer.

Day 18

BREAKFAST

- Gut-Friendly Smoothie

Although fasting helps to reduce inflammation by itself, adding turmeric to your diet can further boost the effect. The main compound in turmeric, curcumin, has been shown to have an important anti-inflammatory effect.

Ingredients

- 1 cup canned unsweetened full-fat coconut milk

- 1 tablespoon coconut oil

- 1 tablespoon chia seeds

- ½ ripe medium banana

- ½ teaspoon ground turmeric

- ½ teaspoon ground cinnamon

Preparation

- Mix all the ingredients in a blender properly, and enjoy afterwards.

•Chicken with Sautéed Tomatoes and Pine Nuts

In an ordinary dish, sautéed tomatoes and pine nuts add a nice nutty flavor. You can also add this topping to fish or beef.

Ingredients

- ¼ cup olive oil

- 1 cup halved cherry tomatoes

- ¼ cup green chilies, chopped

- ¼ cup fresh cilantro

- ½ cup pine nuts

- 2 boneless skinless chicken breasts

Preparation

- Steam the olive oil over medium to high steam for 30 seconds in a medium skillet. Fry tomatoes, chilies, cilantro and pine nuts for about 5 minutes until golden brown. Set aside.

•Cook chicken on each side in the same saucepan for 5
minutes.

•Bring the tomato paste back into the pan and seal.
Simmer over low for 5 minutes until the chicken is
completely cooked.

DINNER

•Mini frittatas

Ingredients

•6 eggs

•1 cup chopped spinach

•12 cherry tomatoes, halved

•1/3 cup diced red bell pepper

•1/3 cup diced green bell pepper

•½ cup green onions, finely chopped

•½ cup grated cheddar cheese (about 2 ounces), plus more
for topping (this is optional)

•1 tablespoon Himalayan salt

•1 teaspoon freshly ground black pepper

•6 slices bacon

Prep time: 15 minutes

Cook time: 20 minutes

Yield: 6 frittatas (2 to 3 servings)

Preparation

•Oven preheat to 300 ° F. Grease the butter or coconut oil into a 6-cup muffin tin.

•Combine the potatoes, spinach, carrots, bell peppers, green onions, cheese, salt, and pepper together in a medium sized dish.

•Wrap a bacon strip around the inside of each cup of muffins. Trim it, and add it to the egg mix if there is any left.

•Fill the egg mixture with every muffin cup about three-quarters full. Cheese top (if used).

•Put and bake in the oven for 20 minutes or until the tops are golden.

•Remove from the oven and allow to cool for 10 minutes.

Day 19

BREAKFAST

- Pineapple Turmeric Smoothie

This yummy, anti-inflammatory smoothie on the stomach is refreshing, smooth and easy so it's a great way to break your morning fast.

Ingredients

- 1 cup coconut water

- 6 ice cubes (approximately 1/2 cup)

- 1 cup chopped fresh pineapple

- ½ teaspoon ground turmeric

- ½ teaspoon ground cinnamon

- ¼ teaspoon freshly ground black pepper

- 1 tablespoon chia seeds

- 1 tablespoon shredded unsweetened coconut

- ¼ teaspoon freshly grated ginger

•Juice of ½ medium lime

Preparation

•Place ice and coconut water in a blender. Stir in remaining ingredients and blend until smooth. Remove more ice if you like. Serve straightaway.

LUNCH

•Butter Lettuce Salad with Poached Eggs and Bacon

This Butter Lettuce Salad is the perfect light lunch to enjoy during your feeding time. This provides plenty of protein to keep you full, but after fasting this won't weigh you down.

Ingredients

•4 slices thick-cut, no-sugar-added nitrate-free bacon

•1 tablespoon freshly squeezed lemon juice

•2 teaspoons Dijon mustard

•2 tablespoons extra-virgin olive oil

•½ teaspoon freshly ground black pepper

•3 cups water

•1 tablespoon rice wine vinegar

•4 large eggs

•4 cups butter lettuce leaves

Preparation

•Preheat oven to about 400 ° F.

•Line a parchment-paper rimmed baking sheet and put
    bacon on top of paper. Bake for 18 minutes until the
    baking sheet is crisp and crispy, turning once in the
    center. Drain strips of bacon onto a tray filled with
    paper towel. Let it cool for 5 minutes. Chop the bacon
    into 1/2 ' bits until cool enough to handle.

•Mix the lemon juice, mustard, butter and pepper together
    in a small bowl. Combine well. Heat well.

•In a large saucepan, add cold water until at least 4' of
    water is in. Add vinegar over medium heat and bring to
    a boil, then reduce to low heat.

•Crack 1 egg in tight, shallow bowl. Continually stir water
    into a saucepan to create a whirlpool. Pour eggs softly
    into glass. Cook the egg for about 4 minutes until solid.
    Take one slotted spoon from the bath. Skim off any
    remaining water foams. Continue of eggs left over.

•Put the lettuce and bacon into a large salad tub. Pour over dressing with lemon-mustard. Toss to combine well. Divide it between four plates. Attach one egg softly to each platter and eat.

DINNER

•Grain-free pancakes

Ingredients

•2 eggs

•½ cup heavy whipping cream (at least 35% fat), plus more for topping (this is optional)

•1 teaspoon vanilla extract

•½ tablespoon organic honey or erythritol

•¼ cup coconut flour

•½ teaspoon baking soda

•¼ teaspoon Himalayan salt

•1 tablespoon butter or coconut oil, plus more for topping (this is optional)

•Ground cinnamon, for topping (this is optional)

Prep time: 10 minutes

Cook time: 30 minutes

Yield: 4 to 6 pancakes (about 2 servings)

Preparation

•Preheat a skillet over medium heat or griddle.

•Pour the milk, sugar, vanilla, and honey into a small bowl.

•Combine the coconut flour, baking soda, and salt in a separate medium sized bowl.

•Slowly add the wet ingredients to the dry ingredients.

•Heat the pan with butter.

•To form pancakes about 3 inches in diameter, pour in two or three tablespoons of batter.

•Cook at each side for 2 to 3 minutes, until golden brown. Continue with extra bread.

•Top the whipped cream, sugar and/or cinnamon pancakes if you like.

Day 20

BREAKFAST

- Breakfast Salad

Salad isn't just for lunch and dinner anymore. You can enjoy this filling dish around the clock!

Ingredients

- 3 cups fresh baby spinach

- 4 large eggs, hard-boiled, peeled, and quartered

- 2 slices nitrate- and nitrite-free bacon, cooked and chopped

- ½ cup sliced cucumber

- ½ medium avocado, peeled, pitted, and diced

- ½ medium apple, cored and sliced

- Juice of ½ medium lemon

Preparation

•Arrange spinach leaves with eggs and bacon over a plate on top. Stir in the salad with cucumber, avocado and apple slices.

•Add fresh lemon juice on lettuce. Serve straightaway.

LUNCH

•Zesty Pecan, Chicken, and Grape Salad

Coating your chicken with nuts adds a crispy skin which keeps the breast moist and tender inside.

Ingredients

•¼ cup chopped pecans

•1 teaspoon chili powder

•¼ cup extra-virgin olive oil

•6 boneless, skinless chicken breasts (about 11/2 pounds)

•6 cups salad greens, torn into bite-sized pieces

•1½ cups sliced white grapes

Preparation

•Preheat oven to about 400 ° F.

•Combine the sliced nuts and chili powder in a mixer. Pour in the oil as mixer works. Bring in a shallow bowl when the mixture is fully mixed.

•Brush chicken with pecan mixture and put in a 9' or 13' unfrozen baking dish on the rack. Roast the chicken for 50 minutes before thoroughly cooked. Remove from the oven and allow to cool for 5 minutes, then slice thinly.

•Fan chicken on six plates over greens, and scatter with sliced grapes.

DINNER

•Essential bone broth

Ingredients

•6 parts of water

•2 tablespoons of raw, unfiltered apple cider vinegar

•2 pounds of animal bones (it can be chicken, turkey, beef, pork, fish, or others.)

•1 coarsely chopped onion

- •3 coarsely chopped carrots

- •10 coarsely chopped stalks celery

- •1 coarsely chopped red bell pepper

- •1 coarsely chopped green bell pepper

- •1 tablespoon of Himalayan salt

- •1 tablespoon of black peppercorns

- •Other herbs or spices (this is optional)

It takes 10 minutes to prepare.

It takes 4 to 48 hours to cook. It depends on the kind of bones used.

It yields 6 parts

Preparation

- •Put 6 parts of cold water in a stockpot.

- •Mix vinegar with the cold water.

- •Put the bones into the water-vinegar mixture and leave it for 30 minutes. While the bones are getting soft, prepare your vegetable.

•In a pot, add the onion, carrots, celery, bell peppers, salt, pepper, and any other herbs or dried spices if using.

•Put over medium - high heat and heat up the water until it almost bubbles, then heat down. For fish bones, let the broth boil for 4 to 8 hours; for poultry bones for 18 to 24 hours; or for beef or pork bones for 24 to 48 h.

•Remove some fresh herbs while 30 minutes are left to prepare (if using).

•Remove from heat for 30 minutes and let it cool. Then strain the beef, bones and vegetables.

•Frozen in pots, ice cube trays or muffin tins for up to 5 days in the refrigerator. You can also store 3 to 4 months in the freezer.

Day 21

BREAKFAST

- Bacon and Vegetable Omelet

Bacon and eggs are a staple in breakfast. This omelet combines the two favorite breakfasts with vegetables to help optimize your intake of micronutrients during feeding times.

Ingredients

- 6 slices nitrate- and nitrite-free bacon, diced

- 1 medium yellow summer squash, chopped

- 1 cup white mushrooms, sliced

- 1 medium zucchini, chopped

- ¼ cup fresh basil leaves, chopped

- 2 tablespoons olive oil

- 8 large eggs, beaten

Preparation

•Cook bacon in a large saute pan until crispy, about 5 minutes. Add vegetables and basil to the oven, and sauté for about 8 minutes until tender.

•In a second oven, heat the olive oil over medium heat, around 1 minute.

•Add the eggs to the second saucepan and boil for 3 minutes.

•Put the mixture of vegetables and bacon on half of the eggs and fold over half to enclose the filling. Serve.

LUNCH

•Curried Shrimp with Vegetables

This recipe is wonderful as described, and easy to modify to make cooking much simpler with anything you have on hand. You should change the chicken or beef shrimps, and use any veggies you want.

Ingredients

•2 tablespoons olive oil

•1 tablespoon green curry powder

•1 pound shrimp, peeled and deveined

•1 (12-ounce) bag frozen broccoli florets

•4 large carrots, peeled and sliced

•1 (8-ounce) can unsweetened full-fat coconut milk

Preparation

•Warm olive oil and green curry powder 1 minute in a large medium heat pan.

•Fill the skillet with steak, broccoli, carrots and milk. Cook until vegetables are tender and about 15 minutes of milk has a rich, pastelike consistency. Serve hot.

DINNER

•Pepper Steak

This zesty steak can be combined with a simple garden salad for a complete, balanced meal that is easy to prepare, and full of nutrients.

Ingredients

•2 (6-ounce) New York sirloins, sliced into thin strips

•1 cup coconut aminos

•4 garlic cloves, peeled and chopped

•1 (1') knob ginger, peeled and sliced

•2 medium shallots, diced

•10 mini sweet peppers, seeded and sliced

•2 teaspoons freshly cracked black peppercorns

•½ teaspoon sea salt

•2 tablespoons olive oil

•2 cups cooked brown rice

Preparation

•20 minutes of marinating steak strips in coconut amino.

•Cook the garlic, ginger, shallots, sweet peppers and olive oil seasonings for 5 minutes in a large saute pan over medium heat.

•Stir in steak strips and cook for 3 minutes. Flip the strips and simmer for another 3 minutes.

•From fire extract steak strips and peppers and drain excess oils. Serve foods with brown rice over water.

Conclusion

Congratulations. You have mastered intermittent fasting. You have lost weight, you feel better, you look fabulous and you have abundant energy.

It's a hard fact that it can really be harder to maintain that weight loss than to lose that weight first. It can be all-too easy to go back to your old, bad eating habits.

And as you've seen in this book, intermittent fasting will improve your life tenfold in. These are some of the positives of intermittent fasting:

•Helping you lose weight and stomach fat and this is scientifically proven.

•It can improve your health—it can help prevent diabetes and heart attacks.

•It can also help to prevent illnesses and to support you in the long run.

•Maintains balanced brain.

•What's more, it can let you live longer.

There are many different diets to choose from, and whatever time of day you're busy, you can fit the fasting in to suit your lifestyle.

There will be moments when you find it difficult and when you want to give up there will be times, and this is the safest time to seek guidance from others who have been through the same thing.